AF556026

| HARE KRISHNA |

Fodder Production and Principles of Animal Nutrition

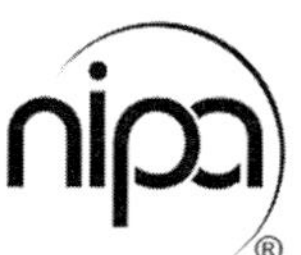

NIPA® GENX ELECTRONIC RESOURCES & SOLUTIONS P. LTD.
New Delhi-110 034

About the Author

Dr. Raman Rao was awarded with the "Sir Stapledon's Commonwealth Fellowship" of England to carryout Post – Doctoral research at Dairy and Swine Research and Development Centre, Lennoxville (Quėbec), Canada. He visited Boston (U.S.); Zürich, Interlaken, Jungfraujoch, Luzerne [Switzerland]; Singen (Hohentwiel, Germany); Bon Accueil, Port Louis (Mauritius); Budapest (Hungary); Bangkok (Thailand) and observed some cow barns, as being a patron – member of "International Society for Krishna Consciousness". He was recipient of a project from Indian Council of Agricultural Research, as Principal Investigator on "Bypassing dietary fats from biohydrogenation for improving product quality in ruminants". He guided and co – guided Post – Graduate students as well as taught for over three decades. He was a member of "Academic Council" of G.B.Pant University, which is known as Herbinger of Green Revolution.

| HARE KRISHNA |

Fodder Production and Principles of Animal Nutrition

Raman Rao
Post-Doctoral Research Fellow [Canada]
Department of Animal Nutrition
College of Veterinary and Animal Science
G B Pant University of Agriculture & Technology
Sant Udham Singh Nagar, Pantnagar
Uttarakhand – 263145, India

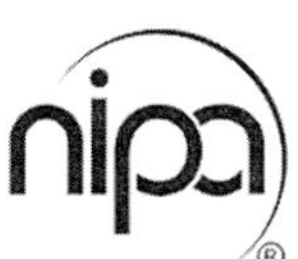

NIPA® GENX ELECTRONIC RESOURCES & SOLUTIONS P. LTD.
New Delhi-110 034

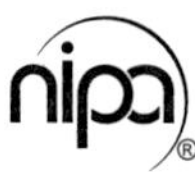

NIPA® GENX ELECTRONIC RESOURCES & SOLUTIONS P. LTD.

101,103, Vikas Surya Plaza, CU Block
L.S.C.Market, Pitam Pura, New Delhi-110 034
Ph : +91 11 4386 0225, 9717133558, 9540816132
E-mail: newindiapublishingagency@gmail.com
Website: www.niparesources.com

Print ISBN: 978-93-58872-43-9

ebook ISBN: 978-93-58874-44-0

NIPA® also publishes books in a variety of electronic formats. Some content that appears in print may not be available in electronic books, and vice versa

Composed and Designed by NIPA®.

Dr. Narendra Singh Jadon
Dean
College of Veterinery &
Animal Sciences

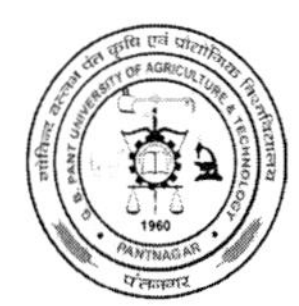

Govind Ballabh Pant University
Of Agriculture & Technology
Pantnagar- 263145 (Uttarakhand) INDIA

Ref.Ne.VlSc/ ... Dated: ....

Foreword

The field of biological sciences and engineering is rapidly growing; and new approaches to solve existing problems are being conceived and developed into new technologies. This book attempts to compile recent developments in the field of food science and animal nutrition. It covers applications of bactofugation, microfiltration, thermization, ultra sonication, microwave technology, hurdle technology, premix formulation, bio-hydrogenation prevention, irradiation and other recent techniques useful in animal feed processing. The organization of book is flexible and allows for individual preferences in the order of study. The authors has blended his practical experience with professional knowledge in documenting this manuscript. The presentation of subject matter is commendable and he has very ably brought together valuable, but widely dispersed, information in this book. The author has fully justified the necessary information in such a way that, it can be used effectively by readers of all skill levels and background. The compilation of varied aspects would be informative and useful in practical field conditions. I am sure that the book will be well received by students, scholars, para-researchers professional, entrepreneurs and academicians. I compliment the authors for his noble attempt in bringing about this piece of work.

I wish all success for the author in the pursuit of his knowledge, and best wishes and happy reading, for the users of this book.

(N.S. Jadon)

Tel: 05944-233347 (0) Fax- 233473, E-mail: dean.vaspgr@gmail.com

Preface

When selecting the theme for this manuscript writing, it was always tried to choose a subject that cuts across as many disciplinary borders as possible. Such subjects are not superior to those more highly specialized, but they are less easily accepted at first. Specialists of any field will always manage to meet and exchange views on their common pet subjects, whereas in the majority of situations, physicists will seldom meet chemists, who in turn will seldom meet biologists, who etcetera ....

Unless there is some prodding from a group in which physicists, chemists and biologists alike are on an equal footing. To compel people from different but overlapping disciplines to meet, is to ensure the cross – fertilization as often mentioned, and which so often remains wishful thinking. It has been said of one person, that if all the things he did were written down, "even the whole world would not have room for all the books". Author doesn't suggest that this is so great a subject, but there do seem to be endless papers progressing at an advancing pace on such topics. Each paper is also becoming narrower in its field, with complication that is designed to keep off all would – be contenders.

In preparing this manuscript, the general framework and character of book established by seniors, have been preserved. The literature survey has been made on the basis of their usefulness to those students who are the principal users of the text.

Suggestions received from teachers, including many former students are greatly acknowledged. The author would welcome suggestions and healthy criticisms for future improvement.

Author

Contents

Theory

Practicals

Theory

1

Animal Nutrition History

Historical Aspects: Eighteenth Century: Antoine Lavoisier, a French scientist was known to be as 'Founder of science of nutrition'. He established chemical basis of nutrition in his respiration experiments and introduced balance, thermometer in his studies. Along with Laplace, he designed a calorimeter through which it was demonstrated that respiration is the essential source of body heat. Even they started realizing that something is there like – carbohydrate, protein, fat and a need was felt for their investigation. But due to bad luck, French revolution took place and Lavoisier's career was ended by **Guillotine (be – heading)**. As a result, further studies on nutrition suffered a setback for several years.

Second half of 19th century: Babcock, an American dairy scientist observed that feeds of different sources were eaten by animals, but there was 'no way of knowing', what particular contribution each of those feeds was making to animal's needs. Therefore, he conceived the idea of trying the rations made up of entirely from a **'single plant'**. He was criticized that his research was highly impractical. Later, his younger colleagues pursued this idea in another experiment. They planned their experiment more meticulously with a greater number of animals by feeding single crop rations. But at that time, they couldn't conclude irrespective of their exhaustive chemical studies of feeds, excreta, tissues of dead calves. It was later on that; the new discoveries provided the 'true answer'. Later, based on this previous experience, 'Purified diet method' was undertaken: carbohydrate as pure starch, fat as pure lard or oil, protein as pure casein along with some minerals then known to be essential. It was revealed that there were certain other nutritionally essentials which were very important.

Opening of 20th century: research with artificial diets were repeated. Frederic Hopkins began his career from Cambridge university in the field of bio – chemistry and nutrition. Early in his career, he isolated, purified and identified tryptophan and showed that 'Zein, a corn protein' could be improved nutritionally by adding this essential amino acid to it. He stated that no animal can survive on purified diet only, but there were certain other important factors which were highly vital for animals. He coined the term **"Accessory growth factors"**, which were essential for the prevention of deficiency diseases. For these pioneering concepts of vitamins, he received "Nobel prize for Medicine in 1939" along with Eijkman. Animal Nutrition research in Indian sub – continent: As early as nineteen hundred twenties, a need for animal nutrition research was felt and hence, a laboratory of physiological chemist was established at Imperial Agriculture Research Institute (IARI), Pusa, Bihar in August, 1921 and was headed by Dr. F. J. Warth. In 1923, this laboratory was shifted to Imperial Institute of Animal Husbandry and dairying in Bengalore. Later on, under the chairmanship of Lord Linithgow, Royal Commission on Agriculture, the animal nutrition division at Indian Veterinary Research Institute (IVRI) was established at Mukteshwar in 1935. This was the only principal Centre of research in the field of nutrition. In early 1950s, National Dairy Research Institute (NDRI) at Karnal was established with a department on Dairy Cattle Nutrition and Physiology. In 1967, Indian Council of Agricultural Research (ICAR) had started research on utilization of agro – industrial – by – products. In 1970s, the species wise (poultry, sheep, goat, buffalo, camel, equine) animal science institutes were established under the guidelines of ICAR. That's how science of nutrition expanded all the world round.

2

Importance of Nutrients in Animal Health and Production

There are 6 nutrients which are very important to animal body – carbohydrates, proteins, minerals, vitamins and water.

Carbohydrates: These are polyhydroxy aldehyde or ketone as in monosaccharide or polymers in oligo or polysaccharides. The question arises whether carbohydrate is a dietary essential **!!!** Carbohydrate may not be dietary essential, but it is definitely metabolically essentially. The organic compounds – fats, proteins are oxidized only in the presence of carbohydrates. Carbohydrates are the structural components of DNA, RNA, and some other vital organic molecules. Although less than 1% is present in the human body [**because,** constantly being formed and broken down in metabolism], yet without the presence of this carbohydrate, the existence of living creature is at stake. Carbohydrate in the form of glucose primarily provides energy in the body and excess amount of carbohydrate is stored as glycogen in the liver and muscle. More than 50 % of the energy value of the diet is provided by carbohydrate.

Glucose + 6 $O_2 \longrightarrow 6\ CO_2 + 6\ H_20\ \Delta$ E (675 k. cal).

Lipids: These are important constituents of plant and animal tissue and these can be extractable from biological materials with the usual fat solubles, for example – Ether, Chloroform, Benzene, Carbon tetrachloride, Acetone etcetra. The lipid metabolism is in dynamic state. There is constant mobilization and transportation of fatty acids from the depots. Some portion of absorbed fatty acids are degraded in the same way, while others are combined with glycerol transported back to depots. All these reactions are so balanced, that mixtures of fatty acids in the depots, blood and organs tend to remain at equilibrium condition.

Proteins: In 1938, a Dutch chemist – Mulder G. J. described certain organic material which is unquestionably the most important of all known substances in the organic kingdom, without which, no life appears possible on our planet. He also used the term protein (**In Greek, proteos means the 1 st**) to describe these vital compounds. Proteins are major structural components of animal tissue, just as cellulose provides for the plants. Proteins are components of skin, hair, wool, eggs, feathers, nails, horns, muscles, tendons, connective tissue and supporting tissue, such as cartilage.

3

Composition of Animal Body and Plants

Nutrition involves various bio – chemical and physiological activities which transform feed elements into body elements. These feed elements are **nutrients** which are digested, absorbed, utilized to build and renew the components of the animal body. As a result, animal grows and produce – milk, eggs, wool with the help of energy so produced in the body. After weaning, most of our farm animals obtain all of their feed supply from plants. Barring carnivores, the plant kingdom is the original and essential source of all animal life, because plants are able to utilize the energy of the sun to build substances which nourish the animal. Plants make use of carbon dioxide, water and mineral salts to form carbohydrates, fats and proteins, which are utilized in the life processes of animal body. Thus, plants store and animals dissipate energy.

Compositional differences between animal and plants.

S.No.	Attributes	Animal	Plants
1.	Major constituent	Water	Water
2.	% dry carbohydrate	1	75
3.	Reserve energy as	Fat	Carbohydrate (starch)
4.	Structural component	Protein and minerals	Carbohydrates (cellulose, hemi – cellulose)
5.	As source of protein	Good	Poor (except oil seeds)
6.	Mineral content	Constant to species	Variable
7.	Variation in composition	Less	Wide

4

Nutrition Aspects of Carbohydrates, Fats and Proteins

Carbohydrates exhibit protein sparing action, because proteins are mainly required for tissue – building, that is, general wear and tear in the body. If there is any emergency, say animal is deficient in calories of the diet, then it will use adipose and protein tissues. **It is said that proteins and fats are burnt (or oxidized) in the flame of carbohydrate**. It means that certain intermediary compounds of glucose oxidation through Krebs cycle, are absolutely necessary for oxidation of proteins and fats. Again, in any emergency, if glucose level of the body goes down, fats and proteins are taken over and they get metabolized faster than the body can take care of the intermediate products. However, **ketone bodies** – acetone, acetoacetate **β – hydroxy butyrate appear in urine. In addition to above, monosaccharides are very important (vital) structural components of many compounds which regulate metabolism. Among these are DNA, RNA** for transfer of genetic information of the cell, which contain ribose and deoxy ribose sugars. **Glucuronic acid** occurs in the liver and this combines with toxic chemicals and bacterial by – products and hence, acts as detoxifying agent. **Hyaluronic acid** (a disaccharide) forms matrix of connective tissue. **Heparin**, a mucopolysaccharide, is very important anti – coagulant. **Chondroitin sulfates** are present in cartilage, bone, skin and tendon. **Glycosides** are widely distributed throughout the plant kingdom and a number of them have been used as drugs for animals.

Lipids: these are the most concentrated form of the stored energy in animal kingdom, because they provide 2.25 times per unit more energy than carbohydrate. They provide insulation for vital organs protecting them from mechanical shock and also maintain body temperature. The cell membranes have phospholipids, for example – Erythrocytes. Prostaglandins exhibit hormonal activities. Essential fatty acids – linoleic, linolenic and arachidonic acids show deficiency symptoms in their absence. **Lipid also delays hunger**, because it requires longer time to pass through stomach than carbohydrate or protein. They also help in lubrication.

Proteins: These are involved in communication (nerves), defense (antibodies), metabolic regulators (hormones), biochemical catalysts (enzymes) and oxygen transport (haemoglobin). For wear and tear or general maintenance of the body, proteins are constantly in demand. Lipids and carbohydrates are stored by the body as energy reserves, but proteins are not stored to any appreciable extent. It is possible for animals to survive for a short period of time on a diet consisting of proteins, vitamins and minerals, but an animal may not survive over the same period of time on **protein – free diet** containing lipids, carbohydrates, vitamins and minerals. Proteins and amino acids are important for the synthesis of cell protoplasm. During the metabolism, old tissues are worn out and new tissues are synthesized. They also help in the synthesis of **bile acids**. All the enzymes are proteins, we can imagine the importance. Milk proteins, antibodies, for example – **colostrum (ϒ globulins), melanin** (skin pigment), **rhodopsin** (visual pigment in eye) are of high significance.

5

Role and Requirement of Water

Role of water

Water is the principal constituent of living plants as well as animal body. With the maturity of seed, water content decreases. Animal body is composed of two thirds of water – intra and extra cellular fluids, and that a feed is any substance used by the body for building tissue, it is obvious that water is very important nutrient. Experiments have shown that animals may live for 100 days without organic feed, but they may die within 5 to 10 days, when deprived off water. Cell rigidity and elasticity imparts a definite form to body, which may be changed by the liquid content of the cell. Due to its high dielectric constant, oppositely charged ions co – exist in water without much interference. Hydrolysis is an important chemical process in digestion and other metabolism, where H^+ and OH^- ions of water are introduced into bigger molecules and these bigger molecules are broken down into smaller units.

Lubrication is yet another important function where water prevents friction or drying in joints, conjunctiva, mouth, pleura surrounding lungs, other soft organs. Body heat regulation is carried out due to certain properties – for example, due to high specific heat conducting power, water can carry away heat from the site of production and distributing it throughout the body. Yet another due to such property, highest latent heat of evaporation from skin, lungs or tongue. Oxygen and carbon di oxide are soluble in water, hence gaseous exchange takes place in the tissues, for example, fish. The **"aqueous humour"** of eye helps to keep up the 'shape' and **'elasticity'** of the eye – ball and acts as refractive medium.

Water content of animal body is variable and decreases as age increases. For example:

- A cattle embryo contains 95 % water
- A new born calf contains 75 – 80 % water
- 5-month-old calf contains 66 – 72 % water

The distribution of water within the body is not uniform. Water content of animal body depends on nutritional status of the animal.

- Blood plasma contains 90 – 92 % water
- Heart, kidney and lungs contain 80 % water
- Muscle contains 75 % water
- Bones contain 45 % water
- Tooth enamel only 5 % water.

6

Measures of Food Energy

Points to ponder

- Minerals are naturally formed substances in earth. They are typically solid, inorganic, have crystal structure formed by geological processes naturally. They may consist of single chemical element or a compound more usually. They are identified by these characteristics: colour, streak, hardness, hardness, luster, diaphaneity, specific gravity, cleavage, fracture, magnetism, solubility.
- Colour in minerals: Its result of brain's interpretation of the dominant wavelength of light. "Minerals are coloured, because certain wavelengths of incident light are absorbed and the colour we perceive is produced by the remaining wavelengths that were not absorbed". Some minerals are colourless.
- The mineral is an essential element which has a metabolic role in the body and if not provided in the diet, can cause deficiency symptoms, which can be prevented by adding that element to the diet. Animal body contains about 3% minerals, which are constant constituents of animal tissue.
- Classification is based on the amount required by the animals. Major elements are required in large amounts and are expressed in % age, whereas minor or trace elements are required in small amounts and hence expressed in parts per million (ppm) or parts per billion (ppb) or even parts per trillion (ppt) .... so on and so forth, depending on *discovery of new trace element.*
- They have following significant role in the cattle: health, production, reproduction, defense.
- For ovine and bovine population: they get minerals from pasture and forages they are grazing, since these feeds contribute the highest % age of diet. These feeds are in fact, good sources of most the required minerals.

- **"Hand – feed"** ovine and bovine population a loose mineral salt mixture with copper. Rumen microbes require Sulfur and Phosphorus in large amounts for proper fermentation and a number of trace minerals in low concentrations.
- Clinical aspects: Rigmin forte is popular among farmers. It's a chelated mixture for cattle. Because, it improves conception rate, reduces calving interval, therefore, healthier young calves are born. Gastina is anti – bloat, stomach – tube is for rapid relief. For reducing acidity in cows, reduction in concentrate and increase in roughage diet + advisable to transfer the rumen contents of a healthy cow. Feeding grains and fats would reduce CH4. Changing cattle diets too for gas issue. Allow livestock free – choice access to portions of pasture windrowed {raked up or heaped up for air drying} for several days prior to dry – grass hay, grain or crop residues. While grazing, lush high bloat – potential plants be avoided.
- Caution: Plastics, polyethene are not minerals, because not naturally occurring. It's a solid, has a definite chemical composition. However, its atoms are not arranged in a regular way. They are made from oil (an inorganic material) by humans. Banned.
- Halite is salty, common table salt (rock salt), is composed of sodium chloride.

Importance of minerals and their requirements in animal health and production: Table 1.

Table 1: Metabolic role, deficiency symptoms and sources of mineral elements

Major minerals			
Minerals	**Metabolic role in the body**	**Deficiency symptoms**	**Sources**
Ca	• Important constituent of skeleton, cells, fluids. • Presence is important for the enzyme system. • Role in the transmission of nerve impulses. • Coagulation of blood. • Role in the egg – shell formation of poultry.	• In the farm animals – In young: **Rickets.** In adult: **Osteomalacia.**. [Imbalance of Ca & P in bone formation in the above both]. (A) In dairy cows (lactating): Milk fever [paralysis, un – consciousness]. (B) In Poultry: Egg production goes down, thin egg – shells.	• Legumes, fishmeal • Bone meal, • Oyster shells, • Dicalcium phosphate
P	• Occurs in bones, phosphoproteins, nucleic acid, phospholipids. • Role in carbohydrate metabolism	• In farm animals – In young: Rickets, In adult – Osteomalacia. [Imbalance of Ca & P in bone formation in above both. • In cattle: **PICA**, where appetite goes down. • In dairy cows: milk yield goes down.	• In the decreasing order (plant origin): Wheat bran > cotton seed meal > linseed meal

Minerals	Metabolic role in the body	Deficiency symptoms	Sources
Major minerals			
K	• Regulation of acid – base balance & osmotic pressure. • Important **intra – cellular cation**. • Important for nerve & muscle excitation. • Role in carbohydrate metabolism.	• **No deficiency as such**, because potassium content of plants is very high. • But, excess may interfere with Mg metabolism.	• Pastures.
S	• Two forms – (a) Inorganic: as Sulfate ions in blood, (b) Organic: mostly as protein (cysteine, cystine, methionine, biotin.: Hormone: insulin, wool. (sheep: rich in cystine = 4 %)	• **No deficiency at all**, because deficiency of sulfur would mean = a deficiency of protein, and this is not possible.	• Proteins • Sodium sulfate.
Trace minerals			
Fe	• > 90 % combines with haemoglobin • Rest: (a) Transferrin: For transport of iron in blood serum, (b) Ferritin: as storage in spleen, liver, bone – marrow, (c) Enzyme component: cytochromes, flavoproteins.	• In farm animals: **Aneamia**. • In poultry: egg production drops • Excess iron: P utilization drops.	• Legumes • Green leafy plant materials
Cu	• Helps in haemoglobin formation & Red Blood Corpuscle production. • As a component of cytochrome oxidase. • **Turacin**: a pigment found in feather, wool, hair.	• In general, Anaemia. • Excess Cu: Teart problem, Cu poisoning, may lead to death of the animal.	• Seed & seed by – products
Co	• Structural component of Vitamin B twelve. • Very important in propionic acid metabolism.	• In ruminants: **Pining** problem, where Vitamin B twelve drops, because, pasture would be low in Co. After several months, appetite goes down, weight loss and then anaemi.	• Spray of Cobalt sulfate on the plants.
I	• Structural component of Thyroxine hormone. • Stimulates egg production in poultry	• **Goitre**: swelling of neck, • Toxic level: embryonic death in poulty.	• Fish meal • Marine weeds

7

Protein Evaluation of Feeds

- All **green** leafy materials in nature have Mg, because it is the structural component of **chlorophyll**. Wherever such green colour is there, carotenes would be associated. The colour of carotenes is red, but this red colour is masked by green colour of chlorophyll. Wherever above green colour is there, vitamin K would also be invariably associated. Therefore Mg, vitamin A and vitamin K would be available by – default or what!! {α, β, ϒ, δ – carotene (s)}. Hence, grazing animals generally would be receiving these nutrients. [we humans may also eat fresh green leafy vegetables {spinach (palak), bathua, methi, coriander (dhania), cabbage, knol – khol, capsicum (bell pepper, Shimla mirch) to get above nutrients]
- Vitamins help regulate body functions, keeping the body healthy and promoting resistance to dis – eases.
- Supplementation of micro – nutrients (vitamins and minerals) as pre – mix, have + ve effects on maintenance, growth, and milk production.
- Biotin, niacin, choline improves milk production in dairy cattle.
- Multivitamin tablet = A to Z0NS may be given (preferably natural sources would always be suggested).
- Vitamin 'B' complex, vitamins C, K are very much synthesized by rumen microbes.

Importance of vitamins and their requirements in animal health and production: Tables 2 & 3

Table 2: Fat soluble Vitamins + Vitamin C [Vitamin C has been included here for viewing at a glance, for convenience]

Attributes	**Vitamin A**	**Vitamin D**	**Vitamin E**	**Vitamin K**	**Vitamin C**
Chemical nature	• Pale yellow crystalline solid, soluble in fat solvents. • Readily destroyed by light or air	There are 10 different forms, but only 2 are naturally occurring – D_2 (Ergocalciferol) and D_3 (Cholecalciferol).	There are 8 naturally occurring forms ÷ into 2 groups – (a) Saturated: α β ϒ δ Tocopherols. α is the most biologically active form. (b) Unsaturated α β ϒ δ Tocotrienols. This α form is 25 % that of α Saturated form	• Also known as Koagulation factor (in foreign language at the place of discovery). • Ruminants can synthesize. • Two forms: K_1 (Naturally occurring) and K_2 (bacterial). • Rapidly destroyed on exposure to Sun – light.	• Chemically known as L – Ascorbic acid. • This is synthesized by Ruminants, Poultry birds, hence not required. • Rapidly destroyed on exposure to light or air.
Sources	• Liver (because of storage) • All carotene containing plant sources, eg. Carrots, green leafy plant materials.	$D_{2:}$ Sun – dried roughages and dead leaves of growing plants. D_3: Some fish, cod liver oil, egg – yolk, colustrum	• Green fodders • Young grasses (not mature ones) • Cereal grains. • Animal sources are poor in vitamin E.	• K_1: Green leafy material, Lucerne, Cabbage. Animal sources: Egg – yolk, fish meal. • K_2 = Bacteria;	• Citrus fruits, green succulent leafy vegetable. • Commercially are also available.

Attributes	**Vitamin A**	**Vitamin D**	**Vitamin E**	**Vitamin K**	**Vitamin C**
Metabolic role	• Vitamin A (***trans***) retinol is inactive, gets oxidized in dim light to retinal (***trans***) & then its isomer (***cis***) form. Now this cis form + opsin Rhodopsin photo receptor. • When light falls on retina, cis is converted to trans & released from opsin. This conversion results in an impulse along the optic nerve to brain. • Protects epithelial cells of mucous membrane.	• Helps in calcium absorption. • Has a role in growth, deposition of calcium and phosphorus on bones. • Helps in Parathyroid activity.	• Biological anti – oxidant. • Prevents the oxidation of unsaturated fatty acids. • Acts as hydrogen donor in the hydrogen transferring system.	• Helps in blood clotting for the formation of Prothrombin. • Has a role in Electron Transport Chain.	• Has a role in Oxidation – Reduction mechanism. • Has a role only in man & other Primates: monkey, guinea pig, bat.
Deficiency symptoms: (a) Farm animals:	• Rough hair, scaly skin. • Night blindness • Xerophthalmia (dryness of Conjuctiva).	• In young animals: Rickets • In older animals: Osteomalacia.	• Muscular dystrophy (where circulatory & respiratory problems are associated).	• No deficiency in farm animals. Because, synthesized by rumen microbes. • Moreover all green leafy materials are rich in Vitamin K.	• No deficiency in farm animals. • Scurvy only Primates and humans.
(b) Swine	• Night blindness • Xerophthalmia	• Paralysis	• Fatal sycope (heart muscle is affected, may lead to death of the animal.	• Nil	• Nil
(c) Poultry	• High mortality rate. • Staggering gait	• Egg production goes down. • Imbalance of Ca & P metabolism.	• Encephalomalacia	• Delayed clotting. Grasses be included in the ration.	• Nil

Table 3: Vitamin B - Complex

Vitamin	Chemical nature	Metabolic role	Deficiency symptoms	Sources
Thiamine	Thiamine di phosphate (TPP) form is found in animal tissue	• Oxidative decarboxylation of pyruvic acid • Participation in Hexose Monophosphate (HMP) shunt pathway.	• In farm animals: Nervous disorders, Beri – Beri. • In poultry: Polyneuritis.	• Liver • Yeast • Germinating grains.
Riboflavin	Structural component of Flavoproteins	• Biosynthesis of flavin nucleotides (FMN, FAD coenzymes) • Role in oxidation – reduction reactions	• In farm animals: Growth goes down, eye – diseases. • In chicks: Curled toe paralysis.	• Liver • Yeast • Green leafy crops.
Pantothenic acid	Structural component of Co – enzyme A	• Important in the formation of Co – A • In combination with two – carbon fragments from carbohydrate, fat, some amino acids, enters Kreb cycle.	• In farm animals: Growth goes down, lesions (wounds) in alimentary canal and nervous tissues. • In chicks: Dermatitis.	• Alpha – alpha • Yeast, molasses • Rice, wheat bran.
Biotin	A co – enzyme	• Important for incorporation (addition) of one – carbon through CO_2 into organic compounds.	• In farm animals: Weight loss. • In poultry: Dermatitis.	• Liver • Yeast • Cereals
Cyano Cobalamine	Cyanide radical Cobalt are the structural component.	• Role in Glutamic acid metabolism, certain alcohols. • Helps in the synthesis of nucleic acids.	• In farm animals: Growth goes down • In cattle: Wasting sickness.	• Synthesized by microbes. • Liver (because of storage) • This the **only member** of B – Complex, which is **Stored.**

8

Measures of Food Energy and Their Application

There are 3 types of systems for expressing the energy value of feeds and many examples have been depicted in each of these systems the world over, but here, one example has been taken up in each of these categories.

[a] **Digestive Nutrient Type**: For example, Total Digestible Nutrient (TDN) system: Digestibility coefficients of various organic nutrients like – carbohydrate, fat and protein are determined by digestibility trials, which can be involved for total digestible nutrients as a measure of nutritive value of feeds. Hence only faecal energy loss has been considered barring losses from other channels. Hence, roughages are overestimated by such calculations. Otherwise, this method is simple, economical and has some basis for animals to be fed on such standard. The TDN value is expressed in % age as following - % TDN = % digestible crude protein + % digestible crude fibre + % digestible nitrogen free extractives + [% digestible ether extract x 2.25]. where Nitrogen Free Extractives = 100 – [crude protein % + ether extract % + crude fibre % + ash %] **on dry matter basis**.

[b] **Production value type**: For example, Starch Equivalent (S.E.) system originated from Germany, hence followed in those areas of Europe and takes into account almost all the losses involved in digestion of feed. The method is based on Carbon – Nitrogen balance studies without the help of any costly equipment, but faced some criticism too. The animals were kept in big animal calorimeter, where different sources of energy losses could be determined to the best of their ability. When it was ensured that the ration on which the animals were neither gaining nor losing weight (by measuring the intake and outgo of both carbon and nitrogen), then pure starch, straw pulp, that is, cellulose, wheat gluten (protein) and oil were added to this diet and determined the carbon and nitrogen separately again. Feeds for productive purposes are measured in terms of starch values. **S.E. = Weight of fat stored per unit of feed / weight of fat stored per unit of starch x 100**. That is, amount of feed required to produce as much animal fat as is being produced by unit amount of starch, when fed in addition to maintenance. For example, if linseed cake has

got SE of 75, which means that 100 kgs of linseed cake can produce as much fat as 75 kgs of pure starch, when fed in addition to maintenance ration.

[c] **Comparative type**. For example, Scandinavian system, which is followed in Denmark, Sweden, Norway, Iceland etcetera. This system is purely based on practical method of feeding, where the comparative production of growth, work, fattening is ascertained by means of group feeding experiments. Similar types of animals are selected with respect to age, weight and productive capacity and are placed on adaption period with a standard diet, so that animals may react similarly to achieve uniformity. For experimental period, separate test feeds are included in each group along with a basal ration. One kg of barley (or corn or wheat) is used as "feed unit" instead of starch, which was used as a unit in starch – equivalent system. In practice, comparative feed values are applicable on the basis of actual result and hence, any specific value of feed received proper recognition, in addition to its protein and energy value. Due to diversified farming as well as grains were of different types in different countries, the feed units also differed. Hence, the system was not applicable in other countries including Asia.

9

Protein Evaluation of Feeds

Crude protein of feeds contain true protein and non – protein nitrogen. True protein is made up of amino acids and for maximum efficiency, feed must have essential acids in correct proportion, correct balance as well as non – essential amino acids should also be in sufficient amounts. About digestion in simple stomached animals, the true protein is degraded to oligopeptides (less than 10 peptides) in the stomach, subsequently to mono peptide amino acids in the small intestine. Thereafter amino acids are assimilated in the small intestine.

But in ruminants, the situation is **complex** in the sense that feed proteins get digested in the rumen, but even amino acids are also broken down by the microbes, and thereafter, amino and carboxylic groups are released. **Secondly**, synthesis of new amino acids or proteins takes place for formation of their own microbial body coat. Because of these reasons, the approach for protein evaluation or expression is different in ruminant animal. Further, non-protein portion of the feed cannot be utilized effectively by non – ruminants like swine and poultry. These animals are usually fed with oil cakes, cereals and cereal by products, which are poor in non-protein compounds, however, young succulent fodders, clover etcetera are rich in such compounds. In the laboratory, crude protein may be estimated by kjeldahl's method and true protein may be precipitated from non – protein nitrogen fraction by treating with cupric hydroxide or trichloro acetic acid. The precipitate is filtered off and subjected to kjeldahl's process. For experimental evaluation of non – ruminants: albino or wistar rats, rabbits, guinea pigs or poultry birds are taken. Casein (milk protein) or albumen (egg protein) are fed to these animals for a period of 4 weeks and any of the following methods are undertaken to look for the protein quality based on response of animals.

Nitrogen balance experiment: Here, nitrogen consumed, nitrogen excreted in excreta as well as in eggs or milk are considered. When, in an animal, * Nitrogen intake = N output, it is said to be N equilibrium. * N intake > N output, it is said to be + ve N equilibrium. * N intake < N output, it is said to be – ve N equilibrium. **Protein Efficiency Ratio (PER)**: Here growth of the albino rat is measured in terms of weight gain per unit weight of protein eaten. P.E.R.= Gain in body weight (gms) / Protein consume (gms). Protein **Replacement**

Value (PRV): This method measures as to how much quantity of "test protein" is equivalent to standard protein, that is, how much quantity of test protein can replace a standard protein. For this to achieve, 2 nitrogen balance experiments are conducted – one for the standard protein of high quality, for example, egg or milk protein and second for the test protein. P.R.V. = Nitrogen balance of standard protein – Nitrogen balance of test protein / N intake.

Biological value (B.V.): This is the percentage of nitrogen absorbed, which is actually retained by the animal. For this to obtain, a nitrogen balance experiment is conducted. Recordings are taken for nitrogen intake, nitrogen excreted in the faeces and urine. B. V. = N intake – [Faecal Nitrogen + Urinary Nitrogen] / Nitrogen intake – Faecal Nitrogen x 100.

For ruminant animals, most common way of expression is the digestible crude protein (D.C.P.) values, which are calculated with the help of literature values of corresponding digestibility co – efficient in some countries including India. Hence, D.C.P. % = Crude protein % x Digestibility coefficient. There is lot of variation for the roughages compared to concentrates, therefore, **Regression equation** is suggested in some countries: D.C.P. % = [Crude protein % x 0.9] – 3.7. Protein Equivalent (P.E.): This is followed in some European countries: P.E. = % Digestible crude protein + % Digestible true protein / 2 [Here, equivalent is being used in place of D.C.P. Non – protein nitrogen fraction is given ½ the nutritive value of the true protein].

10

Feed Additives

Introduction to Animal Feed Technology: When we talk about importance of feed technology in relation to animal productivity, feed represents the major cost in animal production as:

Domestic species	Feed representing on an average [% of the total production cost]
For sheep (typically consumes more **forage** than others)	55 % or more
For poultry	75 %
For swine (pork)	70 %
For finishing cattle	60 %
For lactating cattle	70 %

Feed processing includes all operations necessary to achieve the maximum potential of nutritional value of a feed stuff. The process involves changing ingredients in such a manner as to maximize their natural value and the net returns from their use. Feed processing may be accompanied by Physical, Chemical, Thermal, Bacterial or other changes of a feed ingredient before it is fed. The primary reasons for processing feeds are to make changes in the moisture content, density of feed, particle size, palatability; or to make more profit, to improve nutrient availability, keeping quality (shelf – life); or to reduce storage – transportation space, cost, moulds, Salmonella and other harmful substances. **Feed mill equipment:** The milling industry has been concerned with **"Grinding"** – a process of particle size reduction. During earlier times, the same equipment was used

to produce ↗ Food for humans
↘ Food for livestock because, the process was basically 'grinding' of whole grains. As milling developed into the "Modern Flour Industry", the milling process was extended to include:

Sieving	Heat conditioning
Purification to remove the bran and germ fractions to produce modern white – flour.	Recently, mill owners had started to add enriching ingredients.
Mixing	Pelleting
Flaking	Crumbling

Hammer mills: These are used for the grinding of both – grains and forages. The hammer mill consists of a cylinder – rotar made of several plates, which are keyed to the main shaft or axle. Pins through these plates near the edge, carry the hammers, which are attached to them. Outside the rotating cylinder, is a perforated steel screen. The holes in this screen may be as small as 1/32nd inch or as large as 2 or more inches. Hammer mills may be of single, double or triple reduction types, have knives or blunt discs on one side of the rotar to chop the longer stemmed materials, such Corn fodder or alfa alfa (lucerne) in contact with the hammers. **Attrition mill:** These are also called "plated mills", consist of

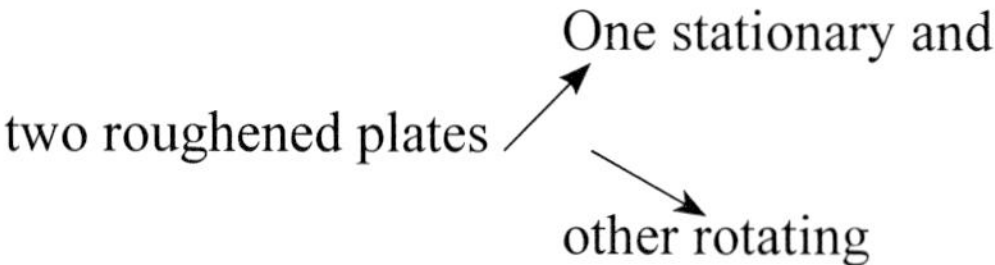

The material is fed between the plates and is reduced by cutting, crushing and shearing. The attrition mill is heavy – duty commercial preparation of feed and food products. Each plate rotates and driven independently with high speeds. In general, it can be said that:

Attrition is more efficient, when producing a **coarser product** &

Hammer mill is more efficient, when producing a **finer product**.

Attrition also produces a more uniform grind than hammer mill.

Roller mills: These are used in feed processing for crimping or crushing of grains:

(a) The double roller mill is used for this purpose, which consists of 2 rolls rotating in opposite directions at the same speed. The material is crushed between rolls. Rolls are usually corrugated or serrated.

(b) The roller mills used in the flour milling industry, have a slow roll and fast roll. They may or may not be corrugated. Such rolls have **"speed differential"**, therefore, cutting and shearing will take place. If the rolls are operated at the same speed, the reduction is mostly by crushing. Roller mills may have 1 or 2 pairs of rolls in strand or set.

(c) **Steaming:** Steaming may be used along with rolling. Live – steam is applied to whole grains in a conditioner. A holding period may be used. A more uniform product with some fines can be produced in a roller mill steam conditioning. The steamed grains are more palatable and preferred by many farmers.

(d) **Pelleting:** Pellets are collected into mass of feeds formed by expulsion of individual ingredients or mixtures by compacting and forcing through die – openings by mechanical process. There could be Hard or Soft types of pellets.

(e) Crumbles, Extrusion, Gelatinization of starch, Popping, Micronizing, Roasting, Steam – rolled flakes, Steam – flakes, Cubed roughages, Feed mixing are some of the other technological aspects.

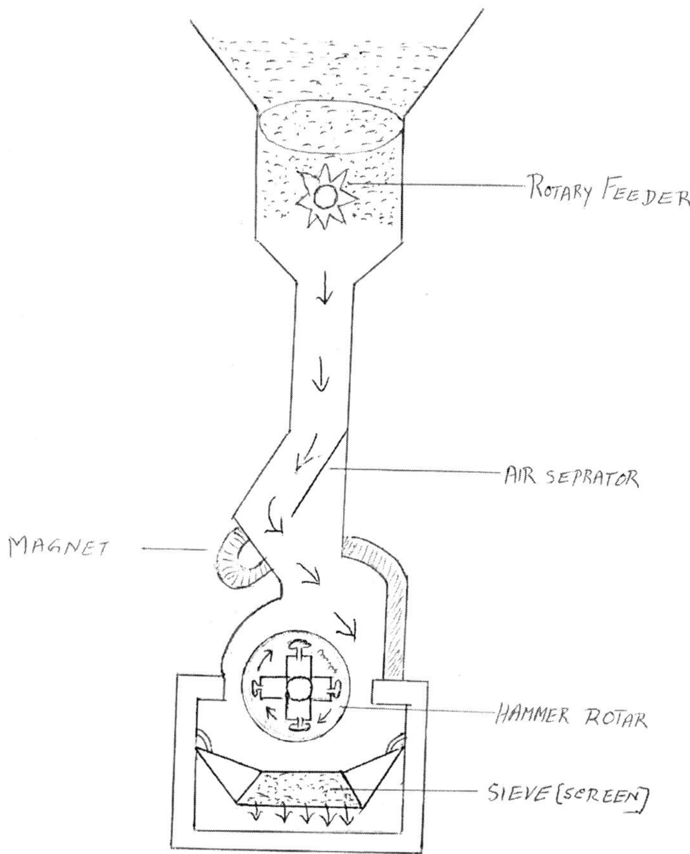

Fig. 1: Vertical Mixer (Diagrammatic Representation)

11

Common Feeds and Fodders

Anti–nutritional factors: Detoxification of undesirable components is very important, because some feeds may contain toxic substances, the excess consumption of which may cause decreased nutritive value of the feeds or may injure some vital organs or even cause death. Some natural inhibitors in feedstuffs are as following:

Feed stuff	Inhibitor(s) or Toxins	De-activating process
Oil cake	Mould	Add propionate, ammonia
Ground nut cake	Aflatoxin	Add ammonium hydroxide, fungicidal
All feed	Salmonella	Pelleting of feed
Cotton seed meal (Hindi version: *binaula*)	Gossypol (cycloprene fatty acid)	By adding iron salts for rupturing pigment glands.
Soybean meal (oil seed)	Saponin (pectin methyl esterase)	Limit amount feed
Castor bean	Ricin	By moist heating
Jowar	Dhurrin	Nitrate & thiosulfate
Brassica	Glucosinolate	Soaking, cooking, supplement with I_2
Molasses	Oxalates	Supplement with $CaCO_3$
Raw fish	Thiaminase (enzyme)	Heating
Egg – albumen	Avidin (its 1 molecule binds 3 molecules of Biotin.	Heating

Points to ponder

- Anti – nutrients present in the diet, either by themselves or their metabolic products arising in the system.
- Plants evolved these compounds as defensive mechanism against insects, parasites, bacteria and fungi.
- Feeds high in anti – nutrients: **Lectins** = legumes, cereal, grains, seeds, nuts, fruits, vegetables. **Oxalates** = spinach, swiss chard, sorrel, beat greens, beet root, rhubarb, nuts, legumes, cereal grains, sweet potatoes,

potatoes. **Phytate** [IP_6] = legumes, cereal grains, **pseudo – cereals** (amaranth, quinoa, millet), nuts, seeds.

- Anti – nutrient in **wheat**: Phytate being the most important among all, reduces the bio – availability of Iron and Zinc. There could be protease inhibitor, tannin, lectin, alkaloid, oxalate too.
- Main anti – nutrients in edible forage and fodders are: tannin, saponins, phytic acid, gossypol, lectin, amylase inhibitor, goitrogen, protease inhibitor.
- Removal of anti – nutrients: heating, boiling, soaking, spouting, fermentation. By combining different methods, many anti – nutrients can be degraded completely.
- Whether anti – nutrient harmful: Generally, they are present in small quantities that they are **unlikely to harm health**, when eaten as a part of the whole ration – compared with eating them as a single compound. Other times, they may interfere with how body absorbs and uses nutrients.
- Anti – nutrients in **potato**: Mainly nitrates. Tubers also contain small amounts of toxic nitriles, which may cause vitamin A deficiency [met – haemo – globinemia].
- **Millets** have tannin, phytic acid, polyphenols, which may affect nutrient absorption, digestion and consumption.
- **Oats** do have phytic acid, polyphenol.
- **Seeds** may have little of phytic acid, lectin, tannin, alkaloid, HCN, oxalic acid.
- Anti – nutrient in the **plant food**: phytate, tannin, lectin, oxalates etcetera in their – leaves, roots, fruits.
- **Grains** have **α** {alpha} – amylase and protease inhibitors, + phytate, lectin.
- **Benefits of anti – nutrients:** They help, protect, treat against some types of **CANCER**, Boost **immune system**. Tannins retard the growth of fungi, bacteria, viruses, which cause illness.
- White rice doesn't have any anti – nutrient or gut – irritants.
- Tomatoes do have tannin, can harm integrity of intestinal cells, proper activity of immune system + nutrient absorption.

- Sugar has no anti – nutrient as such.
- Potato has vitamin C, but missing in vitamins: A, E, K.
- **Ragi flour**: very good after removing phytic acid by soaking. By germination, fermentation, improvement for millets too.

12

Agronomic Practices of Fodder Production

Feed Additives

Feed additives are administered to animal to enhance the effectiveness of nutrients and exert their effects in the gut or on the gut walls. Some of the common feed additives are: Antibiotics, Probiotics, Prebiotics, Arsenicals, Buffering compounds, Anti – oxidants, Enzymes, Hormones, Adsorbents, Organic acids, Flavouring agent, Pigments.

(a) Antibiotics: Chemical compounds produced by other microbes (for example, fungi, and are also synthesized in the laboratory) that, when given in small amounts, halt the growth of bacteria. They are used at therapeutic levels to treat diseases caused by bacteria. In sub – therapeutic levels added to the feed or food to enhance the rate of growth. Modes of action: They halt the growth of bacteria by interfering with their cellular metabolism by (i) Interfere with the synthesis of bacterial cell wall and cause the cell to burst, (ii) Inhibitors of protein synthesis, (iii) Inhibitors of bacterial DNA synthesis, (iv) Ionophore antibiotics – interfere with Na – K electrolyte balance, for example: Monensin sodium.

(b) Probiotics: It's a live microbial food supplement that beneficially affects the host animal by improving the intestinal microbial balance. Beneficial microbes produce enzymes that complement the digestive ability of the host and their presence provides a barrier against invading pathogens [Figure 2].

(c) Prebiotics: These are the compounds other than dietary nutrients that modify the balance the microbial population by promoting the growth of beneficial bacteria and thereby provide a healthier intestinal environment. For example: Oligosaccharides occur natural in foods, such as – Soya bean meal, rapeseed meal and legumes may contain alfa Galacto oligosaccharids (GOS); Cereals contain Fructo – oligosaccharides (FOS); Milk products have Trans – galacto oligosaccharids (TOS); Yeast cell walls contain – Mannan – oligo saccharides (MOS); they are also produced commercially [Figure 3].

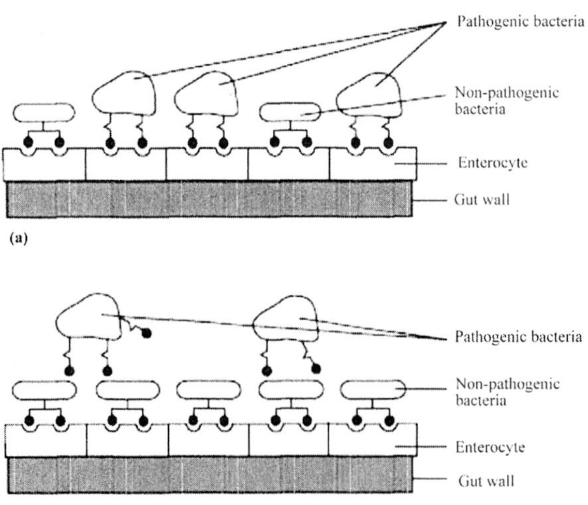

Fig. 2: I. Beneficial bacteria get adhered to the digestive – wall to prevent colonization by pathogenic microbes, for example, *E. coli* II. Attachment is achieved by means of hair like structures on the bacterial surface, called – FIMBRIAE. III. Fimbriae are made – up of proteins: LECTINS, which recognize and selectively combine with specific Oligosaccharide receptor – sites on the gut wall.

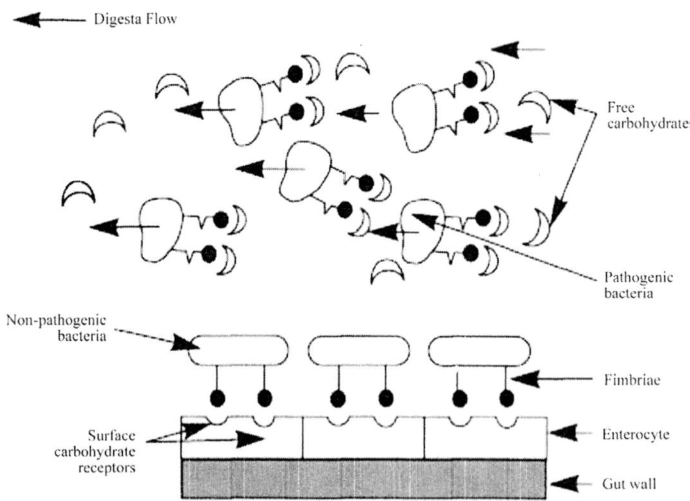

Fig. 3: I. Naturally occurring Oligosaccharides of the feed are Soybean meal, rape seed meal, legumes, cereals, milk products, yeast cell – walls, or even commercial preparations. II. They don't allow the pathogenic bacterial cells (for example, Salmonella, *E. coli*) to get adhered to the gut wall. III. These pathogens are excreted without producing toxins.

(d) Arsenicals: Arsanilic acid, sodium arsanilate and 3 – nitro hydroxyphenyl arsenic acid are also used as growth inhibitors for pathogenic organism and to restore recovering animals.

(e) Buffering compound: These are mixtures of weak acids and their conjugate bases. A more appropriate term would be – neutralizing or alkalizing agents. When present in aqueous solution, buffers should resist changes in pH upon addition of acid or base.

(f) Anti – oxidants: These are chemical compounds which have the capacity of preventing oxidation of substance by taking up oxygen. High fat vegetable products (oils or fat), tallow, lard, fish meal, and poultry by product meal are more prone to oxidative rancidity. They cause off – flavours which reduce voluntary intake and bio – availability of amino acids, and fat-soluble vitamins – Vitamin A and Vitamin E. Butylated hydroxy anisole (BHA), Butylated hydroxy toluene (BHT), Ethoxyquin, and natural anti – oxidants include: Vitamin E, Vitamin C and Rosemary.

(g) Enzymes: Fibrolytic enzymes such as cellulose, Phytase, Xylanase, Beta – glucanase increase nutrient utilization, eliminate toxic effects of feed in non – ruminants. In ruminants, rumen microbes produce sufficient quantity of these enzymes. Exogenous polysaccharide degrading enzymes are stable in the rumen and may pass to lower tract, hence improve nutrient utilization by animals.

(h) Hormones: These are substances produced by endocrine glands that activate specifically the target organ to produce the desired result. Synthesized compounds also have similar response as naturally produced hormones and can be used as feed additive to promote animal growth. They are used to bring desirable changes in rate of metabolism for efficient productivity.

(i) Adsorbents: Compounds that are not absorbed from the alimentary canal and have the ability to bind physically with toxic substances, thus prevent their absorption. The use of adsorbents, such as – activated charcoal and silicates are commonly used in livestock exposed to dietary aflatoxins. Several substances, like – silicates, bentonite, silicon, zeolites etcetera is found beneficial in minimizing the toxic effects of mycotoxins.

(j) Organic acids: Some organic acids especially Malic acid, Fumaric acid are potent rumen – manipulating agents. Malate was found to be more effective in Lactate utilization than Fumarate or Aspartate. Forages rich in malate, for example: Lucerne, Bermuda grass may be used for rumen manipulation. Fumarate was also found to be beneficial for fibre rich diets.

(k) Flavouring agent and Pigments: Flavouring agents are used to enhance the palatability of feeds especially - fish meal and other vegetable protein meals in the diet of (flavous sensitive) pet animals. Pigmentation compounds are used to satisfy consumer preference. Xanthophylls present in yellow maize and lucerne meal are used to produce deep yellow pigmentation in body as well as yolk.

13

Common Leguminous and Non-leguminous Fodders

Common feeds and fodders: An edible material which is ingested, digested, absorbed, assimilated by the animals for their benefit, is known as feed. As per the **National Research Council**, Dry forages and roughages are cut and cured. These are **bulky feeds** with low digestibility. Crude fibre is > 18 % and TDN is < than 60 % because of high cell wall content. Some of the common feed stuffs are: dry grass (hay), wheat straw, paddy straw, oat straw etcetera. Stovers [aerial part without ears and husk (maize) or aerial parts without heads (sorghum). Hulls and shells too. **Pasture range plants**, tree leaves and forages are either harvested or without harvesting (fresh) are also very good for feeding, for example: pasture grass, range plants, tree leaves, green forages. **Concentrates** have < than 18 % crude fibre and > than 60 % TDN. Feeds **rich in protein** (plant origin) are: Cotton seeds / cakes, Mustard cake, Groundnut cake. Whereas animal origin protein sources are: Skim milk, Fish meal, Blood meal. Feeds **rich in carbohydrates (energy)** in grains are: Maize, Oat, Barley. Whereas grain by – products are: Wheat bran, Rice bran, Gram husk, Pulse chuni.

Points to ponder

- Animals are sometimes said "to feed" or to eat, therefore to mean = "food for animal". The old English root is **fedan** = "nourish, sustain or foster".
- **Fodders** are harvested and taken to animals; whereas, **Forages** are browsed on by animals, while still on the land.
- **Feed manufacturing** refers to the process of producing animal feed from **raw** agricultural products; whereas, **Fodder** produced by **manufacturing** is formulated to meet specific animal nutrition requirements for (i) different species of animals, (ii) different life stages. The idea is: to transfer the seed energy and the plant's energy to the animal.

- Maize is the kharif crop that is used both as food and fodder.
- King of the crop, they call is – berseem (clover).
- Fodder making: The seed of desired fodder crop like: maize, bajara, wheat or oat is soaked in water for 12 hours. After which, it is kept in gunny bag for another 12 hours, then put in plastic trays, which are arranged on high density polythene [HDPE] racks.
- Hazard analysis and critical control [HACCP] point system: one has to analyze and assess the risks that certain feed may pose to animal as well as human health + the environment.
- Old English fodder appears to be from proto – Germanic *fodram (source also of old Norsefoor, middle Dutch voeder; old high German Flutter), from PIE *pa – trom, suffixed form of root *pa – "to feed".
- Advantages of fodder are many and **disadvantage = high costs**; because of "intensive use of water and soil".
- Gramineae and Leguminosae families have grasses and legumes respectively. They say, king of cereals = wheat; queen of cereals = maize; king of pulses = chick pea; queen of pulses = pea.
- Functions of feed: (i) stay alive, be active, move and work; (ii) build new cells and tissues for growth; (iii) prevent and fight infections.
- Best fodder – tree appears to be **Mulberry** {Morus alba}. Its high in digestibility, high protein, *holds protein for long time* through Summer, fast grower, hardy (tough !!) and resilient.
- Fodder is important, because it is rich in nutrients and primary source of vitamin A (for, immunity is improved, essential for respiratory tract, and better vision).
- Golden crop appears to be **Jute** for its golden fiber = because of shiny brown colour, most affordable natural fiber and it is 100 % bio – degradable.
- Saffron is red gold, important in pharmaceutical industry. Very expensive and delicate spice, next to culinary function it has for many centuries.
- Silver crop appears to be Cotton (silver fire, cash crop).
- Thirsty crop = paddy, sugarcane.
- Miracle crop = soybean (because of essential nutrients, one of the most versatile food stuff). Well known to Chinese, as traders took soybeans with them on sea – voyages.

14

Storage and Conservation of Fodders

32 – 33. **Agronomic practices for fodder production:** Feeding green forages to animal is economic and better for animal health and production. To get green forage throughout the year, it is necessary to sow the crop at proper time and also to harvest it at a proper stage. According to season, following agronomical practices may be followed:

(a) **Rabi crops:** Berseem, Lucerne, Oat, Mustard, Sugarcane tops

(b) **Zaid crops:** Chari, Maize, Sorghum, Cow pea, Guar.

(c) **Kharif crops:** Maize, Sorghum, Cow pea, Sudan grass, Napier, Para grass.

Berseem and Lucerne (legumes) are best forages for milk production. Berseem is called as king and Lucerne as queen of the fodder crops. Maize, Sorghum, Oat (non – legumes) at flowering stage are good forages. Hybrid Napier, Guinea grass, Para grass and other green grasses are palatable, but poorer in nutritive value than legumes and many non – leguminous forages. Straws and stovers are poor quality roughages. Average voluntary intake of legumes is 2.0 kg; Non legumes and other grasses have 2.25 kg; while of straws, stovers is only 1.5 kg Dry Matter / 100 kg body weight. Following is the schedule for growing of the green fodder:

Crops	Sowing time	Harvesting time
Maize	March – April	May – June
Cow pea	April	June
Sorghum	April – July	July – October
Napier	July – August	August, October, January
Bajra	July – August	October, November
Berseem	October - November	January – March
Oats	October – November	January – March
Lucerne	October	December – May

15

Common Leguminous and Non-leguminous Fodders

Roughage contains > than 18 % crude fibre and < than 60% Total Digestible Nutrients (T.D.N.). **Leguminous fodders** contain more Digestible Crude Protein (D.C.P.). Some common dry legumes are: Pea straw, Arhar straw, Lucerne hay. And some common green legumes are: Berseem (clover), Cow pea, Lucerne (alfa alfa). **Non – leguminous fodders** contain less D.C.P. Some common dry non – legumes are: Wheat straw, Paddy straw, Oat hay, Grass hay. Whereas, some common green legumes are: Sorghum, Maize, Oat, Napier.

Leguminous plants	**Non – leguminous plants**
Description	
These are flowering plants (Fabaceae family)	These are flowering plants that belong to different classes except Fabaceae.
Family	
These belong to Fabaceae family, 3 rd largest family of flowering plants.	Orchidaceae and Asteraceae are 2 of the many non – leguminous families. They are the 2 largest families in the plant kingdom.
Leaves	
These are pinnate, compound and stipulated.	They are simple or compound or unstipulated.
Symbiotic relationship	
They form symbiotic relations with the bacteria ***Rhizobia***.	Many dicotyledonous plants form Symbiotic relations with Actinomycetes: ***Frankia***
Fruit	
It's a legume or pod	They are different types.
Use	
• They are staple food in the human diet, rich in proteins and fibres. • It is also used as fodder for domesticated livestock. • They are used in crop – rotation to fix nitrogen deficiency in the soil.	• Non – leguminous plants can be used in industries, in the human diet, for animal grazing and many more such activities.

16

Preparation, Storage and Conservation of Fodders

Fodders and grasses can be preserved either as hay (dried fodder) or as silage (wet fodder), depending on weather conditions and available resources. These are fed in some (high input) farms to bridge seasonal scarcity periods.

Hay making: * The crop is harvested for hay making at its pre – flowering stage, when its growth is levelling off and its feeding value is still high; * Hay is best made during the rain free days; * Crops with thick and juicy stems should be dried after chaffing and conditioning, which will speed up the drying process and slow down the loss of nutrients; * Hay should be raked only a few times during the drying process in order to avoid the shattering of leaves and bleaching of the hay; * Legumes should be raked in the morning hours to avoid leaf shattering; * After drying and curing, bailing and / or stacking should be done as early as possible. Storage under a roof is preferred; * For hay bailing, maximum permissible water concentration is 15%. Storage of hay before sufficient drying may cause fire due to spontaneous combustion; * Storage of hay with higher moisture concentration may result in mould growth, making the hay unfit for feeding.

Silage making: * Crops and plant materials rich in soluble sugars, such as – maize, sorghum, oats, sugarcane tops, hybrid Napier grass and other grasses are highly suitable for ensiling; * The dry matter concentration of the forage at the time of ensiling should be around 15 – 30 %, but higher is possible; * Chaffing of the material for ensiling increases its compactness, thus eliminates the air space to the maximum content; * Green to semi – green forage, which may use the O_2 present for respiration, results in high quality silage; * The silo should be air tight after filling; * Fermentation starts withing hours after closing the silo, and accelerates over the next 2 to 3 days. It terminates after about 3 weeks. Organic acids, primarily – lactic acid and acetic acid, ethanol and gasses such as CO_2, CH_4, NO_2, and NH_3 are produced during the fermentation process; * Due to production of acid, the pH of the biomass is reduced to a level below 4, resulting in the termination of all biological activities, after which material remains **conserved** under aerobic conditions.

Conclusion: To avoid the loss of nutrients from green fodder at the time of abundant availability, and / or to maintain the nutrient supply during the scarcity periods, fodder conservation can be useful. In humid areas, roadside / forest grasses, and cereal fodders may be preserved as silage. In Arid and semi – arid areas, surplus fodder if any may be preserved as hay or silage, depending on the weather conditions. Leguminous and other slender fodders, such as – cowpea, berseem or lucerne are more suitable for hay making but leaf loss is to be prevented. Fresh succulent stovers of sorghum and pearl – millet and sugarcane tops may also be preserved as silage for better feeding value during the lean season. Since, there are some unavoidable losses in quality as well as in quantity of fodder during the storage, and since additional labour and capital is required for fodder preservation, such practices can only be recommended after thorough cost – benefit analysis. Conservation techniques are a standard practice at organized farms, but whether this technique should be extended to farming families for feeding of high yielding animals during the period of green fodder scarcity depends on local conditions.

17

Safe Feed Storage Techniques and Preventive Measures

For animal rearing it is pertinent to know the technique of keeping and preserving the feed required for the livestock. Apart from the rich pasturage, one may have the longevity of their feeds is immense concern for many. Animal feeds are an amalgam of diverse ingredients, including vegetable oil, sunflower oil. There are also animal fats, like – lard, tallow etcetera, which are included in the fodder. These elements give fodder the targeted input to animal husbandry. The prime factor that occurs and becomes a challenge for many livestock rearing, the cost for their feeds, which would provide quality and quantity in their output. Once the feed is rightly chosen for the animal, that one is rearing, the next challenge arises. Here is somehow animal feeds can be preserved safely, thereby increasing the longevity of the feeds - * Stay safe from the Sun; * Metal cans; * Storage bunkers; * Sliding metal roof bunkers; * Commodity sheds; * Plastic containers or drums; * Re – usable freezer; * Wood bins.

Important dots

- All feed and ingredients have to be stored in a cool place [ideally below 77 ^{0}F or (77 ^{0}F –32) X 5/9 = 25 ^{0}C), although this is not possible at outside locations under summer situations].
- Feed has to be kept dry to prevent fungal or bacterial growth.
- Prevention of entry for rodents or insects is essential.
- Stable form of vitamins is important to use.
- Anti – oxidants are important for preserving fats, oils in ingredients and feed.
- Expiry dates are important on the containers, for all feed materials for their shelf – life (for ground grains = 1 month after milling)
- For fats and oils: Opened container: 1 month; un – opened or stabilized: 1 - year post mixing.

- Vitamin mixtures: 6 months after preparations (exceptions of 1 year, if stabilized with erythroquin). Vitamin c hydrolyses more rapidly.
- Whole grain or seeds: 1 year after harvest.
- Fat free ingredients, protein – meals, minerals have no expiry, as long as feeds remain dry and free from obvious contaminants (these items should carry on acquisition date).

Feed storage area

It's a designated area at the production facility, paved or un – paved, covered or un – covered, that is utilized for storage of any feed materials used to create the rations for livestock. Also included are those areas used to store spoiled, spilled or other un – used rations for livestock.

18

Soil and Water Conservation and Drainage of Water for Fodder

The topic deals with methods to increase the amount of water stored in the soil profile by trapping or holding rain water where it falls, or where there is some small movement as surface run – off. Principles: Choice of method. There is no simple way of classifying methods of water conservation. One suggestion is to do it by comparing rainfall with crop requirements, giving 3 conditions: (a) Where precipitation is less than crop requirements; here the strategy includes land treatments to increase run – off onto cropped areas, following for water conservation, and the use of drought – tolerant crops with suitable management practices. (b) Where precipitation is to crop requirements, here the strategy is local conservation of precipitation maximizing storage within the soil profile, and storage of excess run – off for subsequent use. (c) Where precipitation is in excess of crop requirements; in this case the strategies are to reduce rainfall erosion, to drain surplus run – off and store it for subsequent use.

Some design principles: The effect of scale, methods for crop land: Broad bed and furrow system (BBF), Ridging and tied ridging, Conservation bench terraces (CBT; also known as Zingg terrace, and flat channel terrace); Contour furrows (also known as contour bunds and desert strip farming); Water spreading (the use of run–off areas): Natural run – off; Collected and diverted run – off; Inundation methods, Flood diversion; Surface drainage; Other sources of water: Snow, dew, mist . [Figure 4].

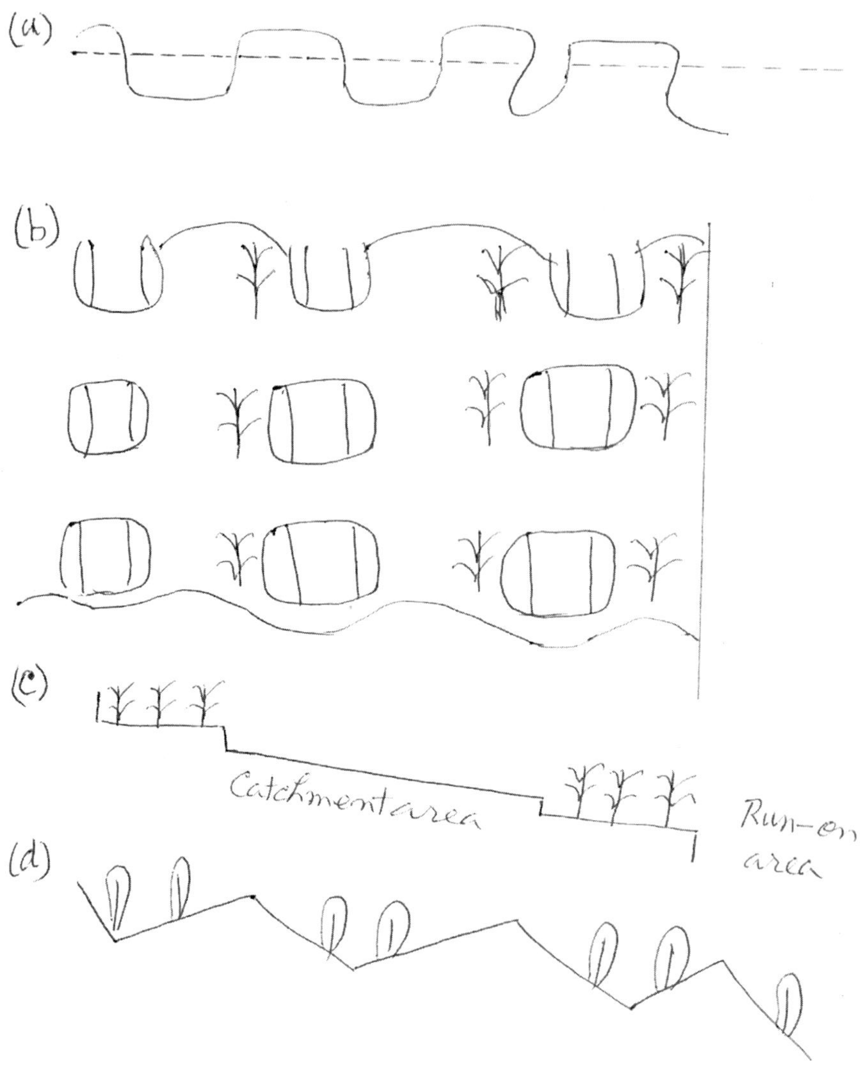

Fig. 4: Methods of changing the soil surface to increase retention of rain-fall on crop land, **A.** Broad bed and furrow, **B.** Tied ridges, **C.** Conservation bench terraces, **d.** Contour furrow or Strip tillage

19

Recycling of Animal Washings and Wastes

The term animal waste comprises, the fresh excrement, including both solid and liquid excreta and urine. * It also includes the bedding material, animal washings, feed waste and straw which are having considerable manorial value. * The characteristics of the livestock wastes depend on fractions of the digestibility, composition of feed ration and species of animals and their physiology. * The waste ruminants have different composition than obtained from swine and poultry, which is having high nutritive value.

For fodder production, the animal waste can be utilized in many ways, that is, as pesticide and that is, as non – conventional source of source energy as pesticides bio – fertilizer to improve soil fertility for sustainable agriculture. This livestock waste can be **recycled** in following ways: Organic mulch, As pesticides, In organic farming, Biogas production, Composting, Vermi-composting, Profitable manure management by livestock fish integration.

Practicals

1

Orientation

Orientation and general precautions in laboratory: Laboratory safety glasses or goggles should be worn in any area where chemicals are used or stored. They should also be worn any time there is chance of splashes or particulates to enter the eye. Closed – toe shoes must be worn at all times in the laboratory. Perforated shoes or sandals are not appropriate. Lab coat, gloves, eye protection, and appropriate attire (impermeable gowns, plastic aprons, masks, face shields) should be worn at all times in the lab. Long pants and shoes completely covering the top of the foot should be worn at all times when working in the lab. Do not eat or drink in the lab at any time. Do not expose electric sparks, open flames and heating elements to organic solvent vapours.

Do not leave your assigned laboratory station without permission of the in charge. Learn the location of the fire extinguisher, eye wash station and first aid kit [A first aid manual, different sized sterile gauge pads, adhesive tape, band aids in several sizes, elastic bandage, antiseptic wipes, antibiotic ointment antiseptic solution like hydrogen peroxide]. Fire blanket, exits from the room, fire escape route. Basic life support (BLS) is important for clinical point of view. Lab safety is important because it can prevent injury, keep us from making mistakes and save lives. Following lab safety rules is part of being a good citizen. We should follow the lab safety protocols to stay safe and healthy. We cannot tell if a chemical is hazardous (radioactive !!) just by looking at it. **Friedrich Esmarch**, the founder of "Modern first – aid". Emergency kit includes - * Flashlight with extra batteries, * Whistle, * Dust mask, * Local maps, * Manual can opener, * Battery powered or hand cranked radio, * Books, games, puzzles or other activities for children.

2

Identification of Feeds and Fodders

Identification / familiarization of various feed ingredients: As per **National Research Council (N. R. C.)**, there are 8 main groups of feedstuffs. (1) Dry forages and roughages; All forage and roughage cut and cured are included in this category. These are bulky feeds with low digestibility. Crude fibre is more than 18 % and Total digestible is less than 60 % because of high cell wall contents. For example: dry grass (hay), wheat straw, paddy straw, oat straw, stovers (aerial part without ears), husk (maize) or aerial part without heads (sorghum), hulls and shells. (2) Pasture range plants, tree leaves and forages; Roughage either harvested or without harvesting (fresh) are included in this group. For example: pasture grass, range plants, tree leaves, green forages (legume and non – legume). (3) Silage; only ensiled forages are included. For example: legume non – legume silages. (4) Energy or basal feeds; Feeds are of low protein content, having crude protein less than 20 %, crude fibre less than 18 % and Total digestible nutrients more than 60 %. For example: cereal grains, milk by – products, fruits, nuts, roots etcetera; (5) Protein supplements; Feeds are of high protein , more than 20 %, crude fibre less than 18 % and Total digestible nutrients more than 60 %. For example: animal, marine, avian, and plant products. Meat meal, fish meal, oil seeds, and their cakes etcetera; (6) Mineral supplements; These are natural or pure elements. For example: composite mineral mixture or specific mineral supplements; (7) Vitamin supplements; These are natural or pure forms. For example: composite vitamin pre–mix or specific vitamin supplements; (8) Feed additives; these are for improving efficiency of utilization of feeds. Number of examples have been cited elsewhere in this book [theoretical part above].

3

Chemical Analysis

Preparation and processing of samples for chemical analysis: The preparation of samples depends upon the purpose of analysis and the nature of the constituents that are to be determined. The preparation of samples for analysis is as important as the analytical procedure and hence, it should be done with utmost care. (A) Smpling of wet material: (1) Plant material; (2) Silage; (3) Cattle faeces; (4) Sheep / goat faeces; (5) Poultry excreta; (B) Sampling of air – dry material: (I) Hay or straw; (II) Concentrates.

Small quantities of feed samples are collected from several locations, all sides, in the middle and are mixed well after chaffing. Such mixture is subjected to quarter sampling, by spreading on levelled ground in circular form. This circle is now divided into 4 equal quarters. Any 2 diagonally opposite quarters are selected and other 2 are rejected. Selected portions are mixed properly and again spread on levelled ground in circular form. This mixture is again divided into 4 equal quarters and any 2 diagonally opposite quarters are selected, while remaining 2 are rejected. This procedure is repeated till required quantity of sample is obtained. This representative sample is brought to laboratory as early for drying in a hot air oven. Dried samples are ground to pass through 2 mm sieve in a Willey mill (large samples may be ground through hammer mill), as described in chapter 10. Sample is collected in an airtight plastic bag and stored in desiccator.

4

Proximate Analysis

Proximate analysis: Weende's system is followed. Weende was a **small village in Germany,** near the University of Goettingen at that time (1860), when this system was developed by Hanneburg and Stohmann. Although it is neither true nor approximate, but somewhere in the middle, that is, proximate analysis of the various parameters for assessment purpose; it gives information about the quality of feeding stuff **and still followed**.

S.No.	Fraction	Components
1.	Moisture	Water and volatile acids and bases, if present
2.	Ash	Essential elements: Major – Ca, P, Mg, Na, K, S, Cl; Trace – Fe, Cu, Co, I, Zn, Mn, Mo, Se, F, V, Cr, Sn, As, Si, Ni
3.	Crude protein	Proteins, amino acids, amines, nitrates, nitrogenous gylcosides, glycoproteins, B – Vitamins, Nucleic acids
4.	Ether extract	Fats, oils, organic acids, pigments, sterols, waxes, fat soluble vitamins – A,D, E, K.
5.	Crude fibre	Cellulose, hemi – cellulose, lignin
6.	Nitrogen – free extractives	Cellulose, hemi – cellulose, lignin, sugars, fructans, starch, organic acids, pectin, tannin, resin, pigments, water soluble vitamins – B complex, C

5

Estimation of Calcium and Phosphorus

Estimation of calcium and phosphorus in feeds: Calcium is precipitated as calcium oxalate by adding ammonium oxalate to acid soluble extract prepared after running a sample for ash. Precipitates of calcium oxalate are dissolved in sulfuric acid and titrated with potassium permanganate to know the content of calcium.

Using $N_1V_1 \equiv N_2V_2$, 1.0 ml of 0.1 $KMnO_4$ = 2.004 mg Calcium.

Calcium, g % = Burette reading difference X 2.004 X dilution factor X 100 / weight of the sample used for preparation of acid soluble mineral extract X 1000.

[dilution factor, (for example) = 250 / 25 (ml aliquot taken) = 10]

Phosphorous present in the sample is precipitated with ammonium molybdate and the precipitates are dissolved in NaOH solution. Excess sodium hydroxide is titrated with nitric acid to calculate the actual volume of NaOH used up which is direct proportion to the Phosphorous content.

1 ml of 0.1 N NaOH = 0.1347 mg Phosphorus

Phosphorus % = Actual volume of 0.1N NaOH solution used to dissolve precipitate X 0.1347 X dilution factor X100 / weight of sample used for acid soluble extract X 1000

[Here, dilution factor is 250 / 50 (aliquot taken) = 5]

6

Undesirable Constituents and Adulterants of Feed

Qualitative detection of undesirable constituents, adulterants in Feeds: The nutritive value of feed ingredients from the same origin may exhibit variation. The factors which are responsible for the variation are natural variation are natural variation, processing, adulteration and damage, deterioration. These days, due to shortage and high prices of feed ingredients, adulteration is one of the main problems. Feed quality can be examined by different techniques:

(a) Feed microscopy: Stereo or compound microscopy may be used for: (i) Screening method; (ii) Floatation technique.

(b) Chemical tests: For heavy metals, nitrates, phosphates, sulfates, free sulfur, salts: carbonate, chloride, salt, sugar, urea, blood, hoof or horn, leather meal, uric acid.

7

Fertilizers, Manures and Agri-Implements

Familiarization with various fertilizers, manure and Agri – implements: **Manure:** * Nutrients are added to soil for healthy growth of plants. * Continuous growing of crops makes the soil poor in nutrients. * Manures are organic substances obtained from decomposition of plants animal wastes. * Manuring is done to replenish soil with nutrients.

Advantages of manuring: * Improves water retaining capacity of the soil. * Makes the soil porous and exchange of gases becomes easy. * Increases the number of friendly microbes. * Improves the texture of the soil. * Replenishes the soil with necessary nutrients.

Fertilizers: * These are chemical substances rich in nutrients. * These are produced in factories.

Advantages of fertilizers: * Help farmers to get better yield of crops.

Disadvantages of fertilizers: * Sources of water pollution. * Make the soil less fertile. * Artificial fertilizers often cause diseases.

Differences

Fertilizer	**Manure**
Inorganic salt	Natural substance
Chemical substance	Organic substance
Prepared in factories	Prepared in fields
Does not humidify the soil	Provides humus to the soil
Rich in plant nutrients	Less rich in plant nutrients.

Conclusion: * Manure: These are organic substances obtained from the decomposition of plant and animal wastes. * Adding manure to the field shall replenish the soil with nutrients. * Manuring results in stronger plants and better crops. * Fertilizers are chemical substances.

Agricultural implements: Hand cultivator, garden shear, rake, wheelbarrow, hoe, trowel, pruning shear, sickle, pickaxe, shovel, axe, garden fork, hose, sprayer, gloves, grape hoe, grass shears, hedge shears, lawn make, spade, trowel, plough, mattock, bolo, crowbar, spade,

8

Silage Quality

Estimation of silage quality parameters: Process of making silage is called ensiling. The green fodder harvested at a proper stage is stored, packed and compressed in silo and it is then tightly covered to prevent the contact with air. Thus, the forage is preserved by controlled microbial anaerobic fermentation in a silo with minimum loss of nutrients for use as a succulent fodder during scarcity (lean) period. This form of preserved fodder is known as silage. Silage is prepared by obtaining enough acid content in ensiled feed which inhibit the microbial fermentation thereby preserving the green fodder. Following are points to ponder:

1. Maize, sorghum, bajra crops having thick solid stems and rich in soluble carbohydrates, are best for silage preparation. Silage can also be prepared from oats, berseem etcetera, after wilting to 35 – 40 % dry matter.
2. Dry matter content in fodder crop for ensiling should be between 30 – 40 % (average 35 %) and should have sufficient soluble sugars for acid production during fermentation.
3. The crop is harvested in bloom stage, which is best for silage preparation.
4. If the crop is deficient in soluble carbohydrates, (for example, legumes), then a sugar industry by – product is added.
5. Silage having acidic flavour and pH 3.5 to 4.2 is considered to be excellent.
6. The crop should be properly trampled / pressed to remove the air out of silo.
7. The crop is chopped into small pieces for better microbial action due to increased surface are and sufficient acid production.

Stages of crops suitable for ensiling

Crops	Stage of ensiling
Maize	Dent stage
Oats, sorghum, bajara	Milk or dough stage
Berseem, lucerne	20 – 25 % bloom stage
Natural grasses	At flowering stage

9

Official Field Visits

- Dairy farm
- Poultry farm
- Wormi compost
- Fodder bank
- Any other visit with the permission of chair.

References

Alkane Technology: Proceedings of the third International Symposium on the Nutrition of Herbivores (1991); Pennang, Malaysia (August 25-30; 1991).

An Introduction to Practical Biochemistry: Plummer, David T. (1979); Second edition; TMH.

Animal Feed Technology: Kundu, S.S.; Mahanta, S.K. Sultan Singh and Pathak, N.N. (2005); Satish Serial Publishing House, Delhi.

Animal Husbandry: Banerjee, G.C. (1999); Oxford and IBH Publishing Co. Ltd., New Delhi and Calcutta.

Animal Nutrition and Feeding practices: Ranjhan, S.K. (1998); Vikas Publishing House Pvt. Ltd.; New Delhi.

Animal Nutrition: Maynard Leonard, A. and Loosli John K., (1982); Sixth edition; TMH .

Animal Nutrition: Mc.Donald, P.; Edwards, R.A.; Greenhalgh, J.F.D. and Morgan, C.A. (1995); Fifth edition, Addison Wesley Longman, Inc., England.

Animal Nutriton in the Tropics: Ranjhan, S.K. (2004); Vikas Publishing House Pvt. Ltd.; New Delhi.

Basic Animal Nutrition and Feeding: Church, D.C. and Pond, W.G. (1982); John Wiley and Sons; New York and Toronto.

Biochemisrty: Lehninger, Albert L. (1978); Second edition, Kalyani Publishers (Indian edition).

Elements of Biochemistry: Gupta, P.K. (1999): First edition, Rastogi Publishers; Meerut.

Feeds and Principles of Animal Nutrition: Benerjee, G.C. (2000); Oxford and IBH Publishing Co. Pvt. Ltd.; New Delhi and Calcutta.

Hawk's Physiological Chemistry: Osier, Bernard A. (1971); Fourteenth edition; TMH.

Lignocellulose Biotechnology: Kuhad, R.C, and Singh, Ajit (2007); I.K.International Publishing house Pvt. Ltd.; New Delhi, Mumbai and Bengaluru.

Livestock Health and Management: Sharma, M.C. and Misra, R.R. (1987); Khanna Publishers, Delhi.

Nutrition and Dietetics under Clinico - Therapeutic Conditions of Pet and Farm Animals: Short Courses of Centre of Advanced Studies (March 20 - April 18; 2001), Animal Nutriton, Indian Veterinary Research Institute, Izatnagar, India.

Poultry Nutrition: Singh, K.S. and Panda, B. (1990): Kalyani Publishers; New Delhi.

Principles of Animal Nutrition and Feed Technology: Reddy, D.V. (2001); Oxford and IBH Publishing, New Delhi.

Principles of Animal Nutrition : Practical Exercise Book; Manohar Lal (1990); Earstwhile Animal Science Department, G.B.Pant University, Pantnagar; Uttaranchal (India).

Protection of Essential Fatty Acids from Biohydrogenation: Where are we now !!!

Raman Rao (2000): The Dissertation of Post-Doctoral Research submitted to "Dairy and Swine Research and Development Centre, Lennoxville (Quebec) JIM 1Z3; Canada".

Review of Physiological Chemistry: Harpar, Harold A.(1973); Fourteenth edition; Maruzen Asian Edition - The Kothari book depot, Bombay.

Text Book of Feed Processing Techniques: Pathak, N.N. (1997); Vikas Publishing house Pvt. Ltd.; New Delhi.

The Mineral Nutrition of Livestock: Underwood, EJ. and Suttle, N.F. (1999); CAB International, U.K.

Trace Elements in Human and Animal Nutrition: Underwood, EJ. (1971); Academic Press; Amsterdam, Boston, London, New York, Oxford, Paris, San Diego, Singapore, Sydney, Tokyo.

Zoo and Wild Animal Medicine: Murray E, Fowler (1986); W.B.Saunders Co., Philadelphia, London, Toronto, Mexico city, Rio de Janeiro, Sydney, Tokyo, Hongkong.

Multiple Choice Question

Q.l. A farmer wants to prepare half quintal of concentrate mixture containing twenty percent protein for the livestocks. Oat (15% protein) & G.N.C. (40% protein) are available in the market. What option should be **tick marked (Ö)** in the following :

a) 80 kgs of G.N.C. & 20 kgs of Oat ( )

b) 80 kgs of Oat & 20 kgs of G.N.C. ( )

c) 40 kgs G.N.C. & 10 kgs of oat ( )

d) 40 kgs Oat & 10 kgs of G.N.C. ( )

e) 40 kgs Oat & 60 kgs of G.N.C. ( )

f) None of the above ( )

Q.2 If "Ash percentage" had been subtracted from hundred, what would be left ? **Tick mark (✓)** your answer in the following :

a) Nitrogen Free Extractive (N.F.E.) minus [C.P.%+C.F.%+E.E.%] ( )

b) Inorganic matter ( )

c) Organic matter ( )

d) Moisture ( )

e) None of the above ( )

Q.3. Heat regulation of animal body is regulated by these properties of water : (a) Very high heat conducting power (b) High specific heat (c) High dielectric constant (d) Highest latent heat of evaporation. **Tick mark (Ö)** your answer in the following :

a) a,b,c are correct ( )

b) a,b,d are correct ( )

c) a,c,d are correct ( )

d) b,c,d are correct ( )

e) All of the above are correct ( )

f) None of the above are correct ( )

Q.4 A farmer wishes to purchase a quintal of Maize grains. Two types of Maize grains -'X'&Y are available in the market at Rs.600/- & Rs.700/- per quintal, containing 20 % & 10 % moisture respectively. What option should be **tick marked (Ö)** in the brackets provided in the following :

a) 'X' type with the total cost of Rs. 375.00 ( )

b) Y type with the total cost of Rs. 375.00 ( )

c) Y type with the total cost of Rs. 388.88 ( )

d) 'X'type with the total cost of Rs. 750.00 ( )

e) Y type with the total cost of Rs. 777.77 ( )

f) None of the above ( )

Q.5 Total number of ATPs (Adenosine Triphosphates) produced after the complete oxidation of one molecule of Stearic acid (C_{18}) would be (answer in code only) :

a) 134

b) 136

c) 146

d) 148

Tick mark (Ö) your answer in the following code :

a) A,B,C are wrong

b) A,B,D are wrong

c) A,C,D are wrong

d) B,C,D are wrong

e) All of the above are wrong

Q.6 Time taken by the movement of egg formation from Ovulation to Oviposition is : (a) Twenty four hours (b) Twenty four hours & Thirty minutes, (c) Twenty four hours & Thirty two minutes. (d) Twenty four hours & Thirty four minutes.

Select your answer from the codes given below

a) A,B,C are wrong

b) A,B,D are wrong

c) A,C,D are wrong

d) B,C,D are wrong

e) All are wrong

Q.7 In late seventies, Dagnela disease in buffalo was found to be linked with paddy straw feeding, which ultimately led to :

a) Skin Dermatitis

b) Disturbed eco-friendly feeding systems

c) Selenium toxicity

d) None of the above

Q.8 When a double - yolked hen egg (as observed in egg - candler) is hatched in the incubator - hatcher, then :

a) Single chick is produced

b) Healthy twins are produced

c) Weak twins are produced

d) No chick would be produced

e) No conclusion can be drawn

Q.9 Founder of 'Science of Nutrition' was

a) Laplace

b) Babcock

c) Lavoisier

d) Hopkins

e) None of the above

Q.10 Suppose, the formation of the first Yolk (follicle) of a hen started on the first day of this month, which led into complete maturation. The fifth yolk would have matured on the following date of this month

a) 14

b) 15

c) 16

d) 17

e) None of the above.

Q.11 Name the Nutritionist (s), who had received **Nobel - Prize (Medicine)** for discovering a very important nutrient

a) Hart & Humphrey

b) Frederick Hopkins & Eijkman

c) Stepp

d) McCollum & Davis.

e) Hoist &Frolish

Q.12 Write 'T' for the true statement or 'F' for the false statement in the following.

If the statement is false, underline the false part also :

* Concentrates have more than eighteen per cent fibre.
* Omasum provides additional storage space for the feed.
* Protein supplements have less than twenty per cent protein.
* Foreign bodies are retained in Crop of the poultry for longer periods.
* Brewer's grains & yeasts are good sources for energy feeds.
* Roughages have less than eighteen per cent fibre.
* Reticulum squeezes out water from the feed.
* Dinanath (Dinbandhu) is a good dry roughage.
* Oligotrichs come under Rumen - Flora class.
* Size of the rumen is eighty per cent of its body weight.
* Yak is a non - ruminant.
* *Copra hircus* is sheep.
* Goat is a bovine.
* Mithun is a non - ruminant.
* *Ovis aries* is goat.
* Mohair is the product from sheep.

* Sus *domesticus* is a poultry bird.

* Camel is ruminant animal.

* Cat - gut is simple stomached pet animal.

* *Gallus domesticus* is swine. Q.13 Fill in the blanks in the following :

* Lavoisier & Laplace had designed .... & by means of which, they demonstrated that.................. is the essential source of body heat.

* Dry roughages used for 'Storage purpose', are called ....

* Babcock conceived the idea of trying out rations made up entirely from .... for his experiment.

* Tallow is ....

* Crab-by prducts are the feed stuffs, classed as ....

* Succulent roughages used for 'Storage purpose', are called ....

* Belching in human being is analogus to .... in ruminants.

* Another name of 'Proximate analysis' of feeds is .... & it was devised by ....

* Lard is ....

* Vomitting in human beings is analogus to .... in ruminants.

* Normal rumen microflora in calf is established at an age of ....

* Lavoisier discovered that the .... was an .... process.

* On an average, an adult cow produces .... saliva each day.

* Cud is ....

* Nitrogen Free Exrtract (on fresh sample basis) - ....

- Vitamin A was discovered by ....
- .... Is the carbohydrate compound in the liver which combines with toxic chemicals and bacterial by-products for detoxification purpose.
- Metabolizable Energy minus Net Energy = ...
- Nutrient .... protects vital organs from mechanical shock and maintain body temperature.
- .... mineral is an extracellular cation.

- .... is the carbohydrate compound, which forms matrix of connective tissue.
- Gross Energy minus Metabolizable Energy = ...
- .... of lipids class, show hormonal activity in the animal body.
- .... is a mucopolysaccharide which acts as anti-coagualant.
- a .... is 25 % more biologically active form than to a ....
- Digestible Energy minus Metabolizable Energy = ...
- A carbohydrate substance .... is an important compound in tendon, cartilage, bone etc.
- .... mineral is an intracellular cation.
- .... of lipid class, acts as precursor of bile pigments, some hormones etc.
- Energy retention is also called as ....
- A carbohydrate compound .... is widely distributed in the plant kingdom and a number of them have been used as drugs for animals.
- Any two examples of essential amino acids are ....
- Deficiency of Vitamin K causes .... problem.
- Synthesis of bile acids, is the function of ....
- Chelate is a ....

Q.13 What was the conclusion of Hart & Humphrey's experiment about **"Something"** ?

Q.15 For which nutritional study, two experiments are conducted ? **Tick mark** (✓) yours answer in the following :

a) For Biological Value determination. ( )

b) For indirect method of digestibility determination. ( )

c) For Protein Replacement Value determination. ( )

d) All of the above three - a,b,c are correct. ( )

e) None of the above. ( )

Q.14 A cow had eaten 10 kgs of fresh Sorghum fodder containing twenty percent moisture and voided 1.5 kgs of dry matter in its faeces. Find the digestibility co-efficient of Sorghum. [Tick **mark (✓)** yours answer in the following:

a) 0.25 ( )

b) 0.81 ( )

c) 25.00 per cent ( )

d) 81.25 per cent ( )

e) None of the above ( )

Q.15 Digestibility co-efficient for 'Ash' is not calculated, because :

a) It does not contribute energy. ( )

b) Pancreatic juice adds more minerals in the ash fraction. ( )

c) Bile juice adds more minerals in the ash fraction. ( )

d) All the above three - a, b, c are correct ( )

e) None of the above. ( )

Q.16 Which Vitamin has the following function? Write answer in space provided.

a) As a biological anti-oxidant....................

b) Protecting epithelial tissues and mucous membrane ....

c) Helping in ElectronTransport Chain ....

d) Helping in Oxidation-Reduction reactions ....

e) Helping in the activity of Parathyroid hormone ....

f) In combination of Se, prevents Encephalomalacia ....

Q.17 Name the type of category, the minerals carry out their following function

a) For maintaining acid-base balance in the body ....

b) For binding with some enzyme ....

c) Bonding of Iron in the Cytochromes ....

d) Bonding of Iodine in the Thyroxine ....

e) Bonding with other minerals in the bones ....

f) For maintaining osmotic pressure in the body ....

Q.18 Deficiency of which Vitamin or mineral causes following problem in farm animals.

a) Pica

b) Muscular dystrophy

c) Milk fever

d) Fatal sycope

Q.19 Write the formulae for the following

a) Total Digestible Nutrients %

b) Protein Efficiency Ratio

c) Starch Equivalent

d) Protein Replacement Value

e) Digestible Crude Protein % of maize fodder

f) Biological Value.

Q.20 Briefly give reasons for the following

a) In the indirect method of determining digestibility, what "assumption" is made ?

b) Lipid delays hunger.

c) Approaches for 'Protein evaluation' is different in ruminant and non - ruminant ?

d) It is said that protein and fat are burnt in the flame of carbohydrate.

e) Lipid is the most concentrated form of stored energy,

f) Calves don't have rumen.

g) Fibrous feeds serve as "Rumen-fill".

h) Foreign bodies are retained for longer periods in one of the stomach compartments

i) Why is it called 'Crude' in :

i] Crude Protein ii] Crude Fat

Q.21 Draw diagram of poultry alimentary canal.

Answer

Note

1. Answers have been given in the descending (reverse) order of question - numbering.
2. For some answers, we have to look in the referred chapters of this book.
3. We should not always ask Google or Wikipedia for information. Afterall, our whole life is a "do it yourself project".

23. Please refer to Figure 2 of chapter 4.

24. Reasoning questions

a) It would be **"assumed"** that the digestibility coefficient of nutrients in the roughages obtained from the First trial would remain the same in the Second trial, where concentrates are mixed with this roughage. Therefore, the total nutrients voided in the faeces from the portion belonging to roughage in the First trial is subtracted from the Second trial to get the remaining nutrients belonging to Concentrates, which would be considered to have come from the concentrate-feed being tested.

b) This is because; **lipids require longer time** to pass through the stomach than carbohydrate or protein.

c) In the simple stomached animals (including we humans), the proteins containing polypeptides are broken down to oligopeptides, which are further broken down to amino acids. And then, these amino acids are assimilated or utilized. In ruminants, all the above degradations are also going on. But, here, **even the amino acids are also broken down.** And secondly, **synthesis of new proteins also takes place by microbes for the synthesis of their own body coat proteins.** Because of these reasons, the approach for protein evaluation is different.

d) Certain intermediary compounds of Glucose oxidation through Kreb cycle are absolutely necessary for oxidation of proteins and fats.

e) Because lipids provide 2.25 times per unit more energy than carbohydrate.

f) Calves have **Reticular or Oesophageal groove (a tube)** in place of Rumen and its continuation Reticulum. This tube directly opens into Abomasum (that is, the true stomach).

g) Fibrous feeds are bulky. The Crude Fibre is **Hydrophilic** (that is, water loving) and hence swells, leading to 'Rumen fill'. Moreover, passage of digesta is also slow.

h) Reticulum provides additional space plus 'Foreign bodies' like - nails, wires etcetera, which are retained for longer periods, to prevent damage of soft organs.

i) Crude Protein = In addition to 'True Protein', they have Non Protein Nitrogen (NPN) compounds, for example - Urea, amino acids, amines, amides, nitrates, purines, pyrimidines, some 'B' complex Vitamins, some N - containing lipids etcetera. Crude Fat = While extraction of sample with Petroleum Ether, some Organic acids, Organic alcohols. Plant pigments also get mixed alongwith lipids in the fraction due to solubility.

21. For the formulae, we have to refer the Chapters-6 and 8 of this book.

20. The deficiency of following nutrients are responsible for such problems

a) Phosphorous deficiency in cattle.

b) Vitamin E deficiency in cattle.

c) Calcium deficiency in dairy cow.

d) Vitamin E deficiency in Swine.

19. Following are the function-type of mineral

a) Electrochemical function (for example, Na, K, Cl)

b) Catalytic function (for example, Mg)

c) Chelating function (for example, Fe in Cytochrome)

d) As a constituent (for example, Iodine in Thyroxine) e) Structural function (for example, Ca and P in bones) f) Electrochemical function (as above).

18. (a) E; (b) A; (c) K; (d) C; (e) D; (f) E.

17. d (all the above - a,b,c are correct).

16. d

15. d (all of the above three - a,b,c are correct).

14. Either, Wheat plant contained 'Something',

Was either TOXIC

Which 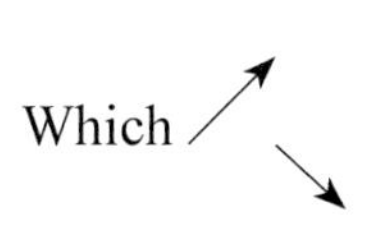

or lacked / deficient in that 'Something'

Or, that 'Something' was **supplied by the Corn plant.**

At that time, they could not name that 'Something'.

[It was years later that the new discoveries provided the true answer.

13. Fill in the blanks

- Calorimeter, respiration.
- Hay
- Single plant
- Cattle fat
- Protein supplement
- Silge
- Eructation
- Proximate analysis; Hanneberg ane Stohman
- Swine fat
- Regurgitation
- Six weeks
- Combustion, Oxidation
- 100 to 200 litres
- Half digested feed
- N.F.E. [Fresh] = C.P.% + E.E. % + C.F. % + Ash % + **Moisture %**
- Me Collum and Margurette Davis (1913).
- Glucuronic acid
- Heat Increment
- Lipid
- Sodium

- Hyal Uronic acid
- Digestible Energy
- Prostaglandins
- Heparin
- Tocopherol; Tocotrienol
- Urinary Energy + Methane Energy
- Chondroitin sulphate
- Potassium
- Cholesterol
- Net Energy for production
- Glycosides
- Essential Amino acids-Arginine, Histidine, Isoleucine, Leucine, Lysine, Methyl Alanine, Phenylalanine, Threonine, Tryptophan, Valine.
- NIL [because, this vitamin is synthesized by ruminants as well as plant feeds have plenty of this vitamin].
- Lipid
- In Greek language, Chelate means **Claw.** It is a Cyclic compound formed between an Organic Molecule and a Metallic ion.

12. All are **false.** Now we can underline the false parts.

11. b

10. Say, if the First Yolk formation started on April, 01st, then formation of 5th Yolk would begin on April, 19. [Because of the following as per the literature survey:

- Two days after the formation of First Yolk, Second Yolk begins to develop.
- It takes 10 days for a Yolk to mature.
- April 1, 3, 5, 7, 9 + 10 days = April 19].

9. c (Lavoisier).

8. d (no chick would be produced, because that was abnormal egg).

7. c (Selenium toxicity).

6. b [that is, 24 hrs and 32 minutes].

5. c [(5 ATPs produced per b Oxidation cycle x 8 b Oxidation cycles = **40 ATPs) plus** (12 ATPs per Acetyl Co A produced in Kreb cycle x Total of 9 Acetyl Co A molecules = **108 ATPs) minus** 2 ATPs expended during initial activation of fatty acid) = 146].

4. d ['X' type with total cost of Rs. 750 /-].

3. b (a,b,d are correct, refer to this book).

2. c (Organic matter).

1. d (40 kgs of oat and 10 kgs of GNC).

Motivational thought

...

Nelson Mandela once said that:
He is never defeated
because:
Either he WINS
OR
He LEARNS

Appendices

Appendix 1: Nutrient Reqirements of Livestock

Daily Nutrient Requirements for Cattle and Buffaloes

Body wt.	Gain (kg)	M.E. Mcal (g)	C.P. (g)	Ca (g)	P (g)	Carotene (mg)
(1)	(2)	(3)	(4)	(5)	(6)	(7)
Growing Anima ls (maintenance a nd growth						
25	200	2.0	120	6	4	3
50	300	5.6	260	8	5	5
75`	400	7.1	330	12	6	8
100	500	6.9	420(275)	16	8	11
150	500	9.1	565(245)	18	11	16
200	500	11.3	580(220)	20	13	21
250	500	13.4	680(200)	21	16	26
300	500	15.6	825(185)	23	17	32
350	500	17.9	985(180)	23	18	37
400	500	20.4	1170(185)	24	19	42

The figures in parentheses represent the requirements for Undegradable protein.

Maintenance of adult cows and buffaloes

300	9.7	290	14	7	30
350	10.9	325	15	9	36
400	12.0	360	16	11	42
450	13.1	400	18	13	48
500	14.2	425	20	14	53
550	15.2	460	22	16	58
600	16.3	490	24	17	64

Pregnancy allowance (add to maintenance) during last 2-3 months of pregnancy

Body wt. (kg)	**M.E. (g)**	**Mcal C.P.**	**Ca (g)**	**P (g)**	**Carotene (mg)**
1	2	3	4	5	6
300	2.8	280	8	6	16
350	3.2	290	9	7	19
400	3.5	300	10	8	22
450	3.7	310	12	10	25
500		4.0	320	13	1028

Milk Production (add to maintenance) per kg milk produced

Indian cow	1.4	100	2.9	2.2
Crossbred cow Jersey	1.4	100	3.0	2.3
Holstein Friesian	1.2	90	2.7	2.0
Buffaloes	1.8	120	3.4	2.5

Fat %	**Based on Fat %**			
3.0	1.0	64	2.5	1.8
4.0	1.2	80	2.7	2.0
5.0	1.4	95	2.9	2.2
6.0	1.6	105	3.1	2.4
7.0	1.7	120	3.3	2.6
8.0	1.9	130	3.5	2.8
9.0	2.1	140	3.7	3.0

For working bullocks

Body wt. (kg)	**M.E. (Mcal)**	**C.P. (g)**	**Ca(g)**	**P(g)**	**Carotene (mg)**
Moderate work (4h/d)					
300	11.1	460	10	10	16
400	14.4	575	13	13	21
500	17.3	680	15	15	24
600	20.1	480	17	17	27
Heavy work (8h/d)					
300	14.0	760	10	10	16
400	18.2	600	13	13	21
500	22.	730	15	15	24
600	25.8	850	17	17	27

Note

1. The figures for maintenance of cows and buffaloes may be used for idle bullocks.
2. For the maintenance of breeding bulls add 1.0 Mcal ME and 225g C.P. to the allowance for the same weight of cows.
3. When calculating the maintenance requirements for lactating first calvers that are still growing. The figures growth rather than maintenance should be used.
4. For cows producing more than 20kg milk per day. requirements are increased by 15 per cent.

Daily Nutrient Requirement of Sheep

Body wt.(kg)	Gai (or loss)	D.M.I. % of L.W.	M.E. or Metabolizable Energy (Mcal/Kg)	(Mcal/d)	Protein Total	DCP	Ca (g)	P (g)	Vitamin A (1000 IU)	D(IU)
EWES and LAMBS Maintenance, Growth, Non-Lactating and First 15 Weeks of Gestation										
10	50	3.9	1.95	0.76	35	18	2.3	1.5	1.9	64
15	50	3.5	2.00	1.04	49	25	2.8	1.8	2.9	196
20	50	3.3	2.00	1.29	59	31	3.3	2.3	4.0	128
25	100	3.3	2.40	2.00	85	48	4.2	2.8	5.0	164
30	125	3.1	2.75	2.57	103	60	4.9	3.3	6.3	199
35	125	3.1	2.75	2.89	177	69	5.9	3.3	4.1	218
Early Weaned Lambs (5 to30 kg) Maintenance and Growth										
5	100	2.3	4.3	0.50	45	36	1.8	1.3	0.50	35
10	100	2.1	4.0	0.84	70	56	2.1	1.5	0.85	67
15	150	2.3	3.8	1.30	109	87	2.7	1.9	1.28	98
20	150	2.3	3.5	1.61	135	108	3.2	2.2	1.70	133
25	200	2.5	3.1	1.91	160	128	4.1	2.8	2.12	168
30	300	3.3	3.0	2.95	248	198	5.0	3.3	2.55	200
Maintenance, Growth, Non-lactating and First 15 Weeks of Gestation										
40	100	3.0	2.40	2.85	121	68	5.96	3.2	4.0	226
50	100	2.8	2.40	3.37	144	81	6.1	3.4	5.0	276
60	100	2.7	2.40	3.85	164	92	6.4	3.5	6.2	330

Daily Nutrient Requirement of Sheep

Body wt.(kg)	Gai (or loss)	D.M.I. % of L.W.	M.E. or Metabolizable Energy		Protein		Ca (g)	P (g)	Vitamin	
			(Mcal/Kg)	(Mcal/d)	Total	DCP			A (1000 IU)	D(IU)
Last 6 Weeks of Gestation or Last Weeks of Lactation										
20	100	4.5	2.55	2.31	103	62	3.9	3.7	5.2	180
30	125	4.0	2.85	3.42	148	92	3.9	3.7	6.5	200
40	100	3.7	2.65	3.90	174	105	4.0	3.8	8.0	230
50	75	3.4	2.50	4.20	191	113	4.1	3.9	10.3	278
60	50	3.0	2.40	4.35	199	117	4.4	4.1	12.5	333
70	25	3.5	2.25	4.37	206	118	4.5	4.3	14.6	388
First 8 Weeks of Lactation										
20	5	5.0	2.35	2.34	105	60	9.5	6.9	5.9	180
30	5	4.5	2.20	2.99	143	82	9.8	7.1	6.8	200
40	10	4.2	2.00	3.37	176	101	10.4	7.4	8.2	235
50	20	3.9	2.00	3.99	209	120	10.9	7.8	10.3	278
60	30	3.8	2.00	4.57	239	137	11.5	8.2	12.5	333
70	30	3.6	2.00	5.13	267	154	12.0	8.6	14.6	388
RAMS Maintenance and Growth										
30	120	3.8	2.25	2.59	113	62	5.9	3.2	3.2	185
40	110	3.6	2.15	3.07	137	74	6.3	3.5	4.2	222
50	100	3.4	2.05	3.48	159	84	6.8	3.8	5.2	277
60	100	3.2	2.05	3.99	181	96	7.2	4.0	6.3	333
70	80	3.1	1.90	4.08	194	98	7.5	4.3	7.3	388
80	80	3.0	1.90	4.51	212	108	7.9	4.4	8.3	444
90	80	2.9	1.90	4.92	231	118	8.3	4.7	9.3	499

Daily Nutrient Requirement of Goat

Body wt.(kg)	Gain (or loss)	D.M.I. % of L.W.	M.E. or Metabolizable Energy		Protein		Ca (g)	P (g)	Vitamin	
			(Mcal/Kg)	(Mcal/d)	Total	DCP			A (1000 IU)	D (IU)
Nutrient Constituents of Goats Milk at Different Fat Levels (Nutrients/kg Milk)										
5	25	4.4	2.35	0.52	22	15	0.8	0.6	0.4	78
10	50	3.7	2.50	0.92	39	26	1.5	1.2	0.6	139
15	50	3.3	2.30	1.13	48	33	1.9	1.4	0.8	169
20	75	3.1	2.40	1.49	63	43	2.4	1.9	1.1	232
25	75	3.1	2.30	1.67	71	48	2.7	2.1	1.2	247
30	75	2.8	2.20	1.84	78	53	3.1	2.3	1.3	273
40	100	2.5	2.30	2.34	99	67	3.8	2.9	1.7	353
50	100	2.4	2.20	2.62	111	75	4.3	3.3	1.9	395
60	125	2.3	2.25	3.17	134	91	5.0	3.8	2.2	465
70	125	2.2	2.15	3.35	142	96	5.5	4.1	2.4	507
80	150	2.1	2.20	3.75	159	108	6.3	4.7	2.7	573
Last 8 Weeks of Gestation and Last 8 Weeks of Lactation										
20	100	3.6	3.00	2.17	92	90	3.0	2.1	1.8	357
25	100	3.4	3.00	2.57	109	95	3.0	2.1	1.9	382
30	100	3.3	2.80	2.71	115	100	4.0	2.8	2.0	408
35	120	3.1	2.50	2.76	117	110	4.0	2.8	2.2	433
40	120	3.0	3.50	3.05	129	115	4.0	2.8	2.3	456
50	120	2.9	2.50	3.61	153	120	5.0	3.5	2.5	498
60	120	2.8	2.50	4.13	175	129	5.0	3.5	2.7	540
70	120	2.6	2.50	4.64	196	137	6.0	3.5	2.9	582

First 10 Weeks of Lactation										
20	-20	5.6	2.45	2.74	116	88	4.0	2.8	4.5	9.4
25	-20	5.4	2.30	3.02	128	97	4.0	2.8	4.6	929
30	-20	5.1	2.20	3.29	139	105	5.0	3.5	4.7	955
35	-20	4.9	2.10	3.54	150	113	5.0	3.5	4.9	980
40	-20	4.8	2.00	3.79	160	121	5.0	3.5	4.9	1003
50	-20	4.5	1.90	4.16	176	133	6.0	4.2	5.2	1045
60	-20	4.3	1.85	4.71	199	151	6.0	4.2	5.4	1087
70	-20	4.3	1.75	5.14	217	164	7.0	4.9	5.6	1129

Nutrient Constituents of Goats Milk at Different Fat Levels (Nutrients/kg Milk)

Fat (%)	Energy M.E. (Mcal)	Total (g)	Protein	DCP	Ca(g)	P(g)	Vitamin-A (1000 IU)	Vitamin-D (IU)
2.5	1.20	62		42	2	1.4	3.8	760
3.0	1.21	66		45	2	1.4	3.8	760
3.5	1.23	71		48	2	1.4	3.8	760
4.5	1.26	79		54	3	2.1	3.8	760
5.0	1.28	84		57	3	2.1	3.8	760

Nutrient requirements, premix and ingredients for surine

Partculars Ingredients	Young		Growing	Finisher	Pregnant sows/gilts	Farrowing/ lactating Sows/gilts
	Pre-Starter	Starter				
CP%	20	20	18	16	15	15
ME, Mcal/kg	3.35	3.35	3.17	3.17	3.15	3.15
Premix (kg/100kg)						
Salt	0.35	0.35	0.25	0.25	0.50	0.50
DCP	1.25	1.00	1.00	1.00	1.50	1.50
Limestone	0.50	0.75	0.75	0.75	0.75	0.75
Vit. mix.	0.10	0.10	0.075	0.05	0.10	0.10
Choline mix.	0.10	0.10	-	-	0.10	0.10
Biotin folic						
acid mix	-	-	-	-	0.05	0.05
Trace min. mix	0.10	0.10	0.075	0.05	0.10	0.10
Antibiotics (g)	10-25	10-25	5-10	05-10	-	5-15
Copper Sulphate	0.10	0.10	10-25 p p m	10-25 pmm	-	-
Total	2.5	2.5	2.15	2.10	3.10	3.10

Ingredients

1. Maize
2. Wheat
3. Barley
4. Rice polish
5. Soyabean meal
6. Fish meal
7. Meat cum bone meal
8. Ground nut cake
9. Fat

Note

A. For preparing meal mixtures for growing swine upto 30kg weight, following are added-
   a) 75% of basal feeds
   b) 15% Vegetable protein supplement
   c) 5.7% animal protein supplement

B. In case of swine having Between 30-50kg body weight, following are added-
   a) 85% of basal feeds
   b) 9% Vegetable proteins
   c) 3% animal proteins

Nutrient Requirements For Poultry (per cent or in each kg of feed)

Nutrients	**Broiler Starter (BSF)**	**Broiler Finisher (BSF)**	**Chick Feed**	**Growing Chicken (GCF)**	**Laying Chicken (LCF)**	**Breeder Chicken (BCF)**
Metabolizable energy (Kcal/kg)	2900	3000	2700	2700	2700	2800
Protein (%)	22	19	22	16	18	18
Lysine (%)	0.9	0.9	1.0	0.7	0.5	0.5
Methionine (%)	0.35	0.35	0.35	0.25	0.25	0.25
Sulphur amino acid (%)	0.75	0.75	0.75	0.50	0.50	0.50
Linolenic acid (%)	1.0	1.0	1.0	1.0	1.0	1.0
Minerals Calcium (%)	1.0	1.0	1.0	1.0	2.75	2.75
Available phosphorus (%)	0.50	0.50	0.50	0.50	0.50	0.50
Manganese (mg)	60	55	55	55	55	55
Iodine (mg)	1	1	1	1	1	1
Iron (mg)	40	40	20	20	20	20
Copper (mg)	4	4	2	2	2	2
Zinc (mg)	50	50	-	-	-	-
Vitamins Vitamin A (IU)	6000	6000	4000	4000	8000	8000
Vitamin D (CD)	600	600	600	600	1200	1200
Thiamine (mg)	2	2	6	6	6	6
Riboflavin (mg)	5	5	5	5	5	5
Pantothenic acid (mg)	12	12	10	10	15	15
Nicotinic acid (mg)	40	40	30	20	20	20
Biotin (mg)	0.1	0.1	0.1	0.1	0.15	0.15
Vitamin B-12 (mg)	8	8	15	15	15	30
Alpha tocopherol (mg)	20	20	10	10	10	20
Cholin chloride (mg)	1400	1400	1300	-	-	1300
Crude fibre, (%) Max	6	6	7	8	8	8
Acid Insol, Ash, (%) Max .	3.0	3.0	4.0	4.0	4.0	4.0
Salt (as Nacl),(%) Max.	0.6	0.6	0.6	0.6	0.6	0.6

*CU stands for AOAC chick unit.

Feed Requirements for Poultry (g)

Age in Weeks	Per Egg Laying Chicken		Per Broiler Chicken	
	Cumulative	**Av. Daily**	**Cumulative**	**Av. Daily**
01			84	12
02			294	30
03			609	45
04	650	35	1029	60
05			1554	75
06			2184	90
07			2919	105
08	1900	55	3759	110
12	3400	65		
16	5000	70		
20	7000	80		
24	10000	110		
30	14500			
40	22000			
60	37000			
80	52000			

Per cent Egg Production	Feed Requirement (g/bird)
0	80
20	90
40	100
60	110

Appendix-II: Nutritive value of common feeds (Straws and green forages)

Class of Forage DM as Nutrient Composition on DM (%) basis Voluntary

Class of Forage	DM as Fed, %	Nutrient Composition on DM (%) basis				Voluntary Intake (kg DM/100kg)*
		C.P.	M.E. (Mcal/kg)	Calcium	Phosphours	
Straws and Karbies	90	3.0	1.6	0.15	0.08	1.5
Green sorghum, bajra,						
S.cane tops,						
Tropical grasses	25-40	6.0	2.0	0.50	0.30	2.0
Green maize	20-35	8.0	2.4	0.50	0.20	2.2
Green oat	20-35	10.0	2.4	0.40	0.30	2.2
Green berseem, Lucerne, Lobia	15-25	15-20	2.2	2.00	0.20	2.0**
		40			100	
		60			110	
		80			120	

*These figures are for desi cows and buffaloes. Crossbred cows eat about 25 per cent more than figures. Heifers of all breeds cat about 25 per cent more than adults.

**The consumption of Lucerne by buffaloes is only about 1.5 kg/100kg body weight.

Nutritive value of concentrate feeds on as fed basis

Feedstuff	D.M. %	Protein	Met. Energy (Mcal/kg)		Fibre %	Fat %	Ca %	P %	Lys. %	Methionine + Cystine	Tryp t. %
			Poultry	Cattle							
Energy Feeds											
Cereal Grains											
High energy											
Bajra	90	10.8	2.61	2.55	1	5	0.12	0.4	0.39	0.18	0.20
Barley	90	10.1	2.69	2.80	6	2	0.08	0.2	0.58	0.38	0.19
Jowar	87	9.2	2.80	2.80	3	4	0.08	0.3	0.16	0.21	0.08
Maize	90	9.0	3.00	2.80	2	3	0.06	0.3	0.16	0.21	0.08
Wheat	90	11.5	2.70	2.80	2	2	0.06	0.4	0.42	0.42	0.17
Medium Energy											
Oat	92	9.5	2.68	2.68	11	5	0.10	0.3	0.38	0.39	0.18
Paddy	91	7.5	2.38	2.68	9	2	0.05	0.2	0.27	0.30	0.10
Roots											
High energy											
Tapioca chips	91	2.1	3.06	2.70	6	2	0.10	0.1			
Factory by Product											
Feeds High energy											
Rice polish	92	11.0	3.13	3.00	4	13	0.10	1.0	0.40	0.28	0.08
Rice polish (Solvent extracted)	92	12.5	2.57	2.30	5	1	0.12	1.2	0.46	0.28	0.08
Medium energy											
Dal chune	90	13.5	1.1	2.2	12	4	0.40	0.3	-	-	-
Rice bran	90	12.1	2.64	2.35	12	11	0.16	0.9	0.50	0.30	0.10
Wheat bran	90	14.3	1.1	2.2	10	4	0.13	0.8	0.50	0.30	0.10
Low energy											
Rice bran (solvent extracted)	90	13.1	2.0	2.0	13	1	0.17	1.0	0.58	0.35	0.12

Protein Feeds **Vegetable Origin** **High protein**											
Groundnut Cake	92	43.0	2.76	3.00	12	6	0.21	06	1.1	1.0	0.4
Deoiled GN Cake	93	47.0	2.50	2.66	10	10	0.23	0.6	1.2	1.3	0.5
Cottonseed Cake	92	27.9	1.66	2.58	20	5	0.48	0.8	1.0	0.9	0.4
Guar meal	90	36.0	-	2.16	12	8	0.48	0.6	1.3	0.4	-
Maize gluten meal	90	38.7	2.97	2.76	4	2	0.20	0.4	0.8	1.8	0.2
Sesame Cake	91	40.0	2.37	2.63	7	8	2.23	1.0	1.2	1.6	0.5
Deoiled Soyabean	90	48.0	2.83	2.99	5	1	0.32	0.8	2.3	1.2	0.5
Medium protein											
Mustard Cake	91	35.0	2.69	2.55	11	6	0.60	1.0	1.8	1.6	0.38
Linseed Cake	91	29.0	1.52	2.66	10	8	0.43	0.9	0.9	1.1	0.5
Low protein											
Coconut Cake	91	22.8	1.75	2.64	12	7	0.40	0.7	0.6	0.8	0.2
Maize gluten feed	92	22.8	1.70	2.66	8	2	0.44	0.8	0.8	0.6	0.2
Animal & Fish Origin											
High Protein											
Fish meal	94	56.0	2.73	2.71	-	7	7.00	2.8	5.9	1.85	0.5
Meat meal	92	45.0	2.54	2.56	-	9	7.48	3.9	3.7	1.35	-
Mineral Supplements											
Bone meal	92	11.5	0.55	0.55	-	3	25.8	11.0			
Mineral mixture (Cattle)	-	-	-	-	-	-	28.0	12.0	-	-	-
Mineral Mixture (Poultry)	-	-	-	-	-	-	20.0	20.0	-	-	-
Shell grit	-	-	-	-	-	-	36.0	-	-	-	-

Source: All the tables of appendix I and II, Manohar Verma (1990); Prineiples of Animals Nutrition, Practical Exercise book; Earstwhile Animal Science, G.B.P.U.A.& T.; Pantnagar (Uttaranchal)

Index